The Allergic Pet

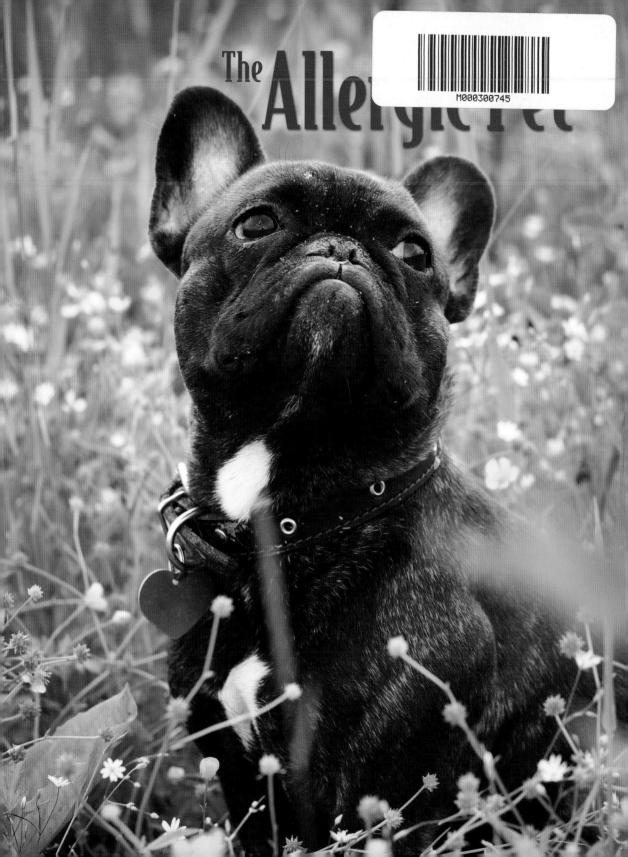

The Allergic Pet

CompanionHouse Books™ is an imprint of Fox Chapel Publishers International Ltd.

Project Team
Vice President–Content: Christopher Reggio
Editor: Amy Deputato
Copy Editor: Kaitlyn Ocasio
Design: Mary Ann Kahn
Index: Elizabeth Walker

ISBN 978-1-62187-182-8

The Cataloging-in-Publication Data is available from the Library of Congress

This book has been published with the intent to provide accurate and authoritative information in regard to the subject matter within. While every precaution has been taken in the preparation of this book, the author and publisher expressly disclaim any responsibility for any errors, omissions, or adverse effects arising from the use or application of the information contained herein. The techniques and suggestions are used at the reader's discretion and are not to be considered a substitute for veterinary care. If you suspect a medical problem, consult your veterinarian.

Fox Chapel Publishing
903 Square Street
Mount Joy, PA 17552

Fox Chapel Publishers International Ltd.
7 Danefield Road, Selsey (Chichester)
West Sussex PO20 9DA, U.K.

www.facebook.com/companionhousebooks

We are always looking for talented authors. To submit an idea, please send a brief inquiry to acquisitions@foxchapelpublishing.com.

Printed and bound in China
21 20 19 18   2 4 6 8 10 9 7 5 3 1

The Allergic Pet

Holistic Solutions to End the Allergy Epidemic in Our Dogs and Cats

Deva Khalsa, VMD

COMPANIONHOUSE
BOOKS

Contents

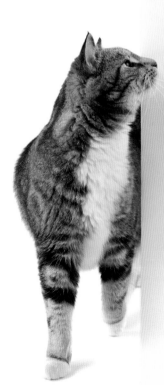

Part III: Finding Food that Works

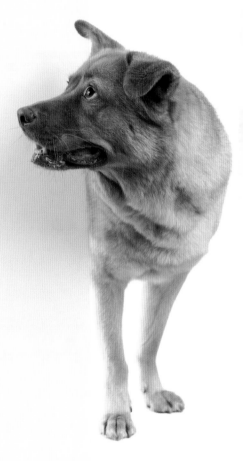

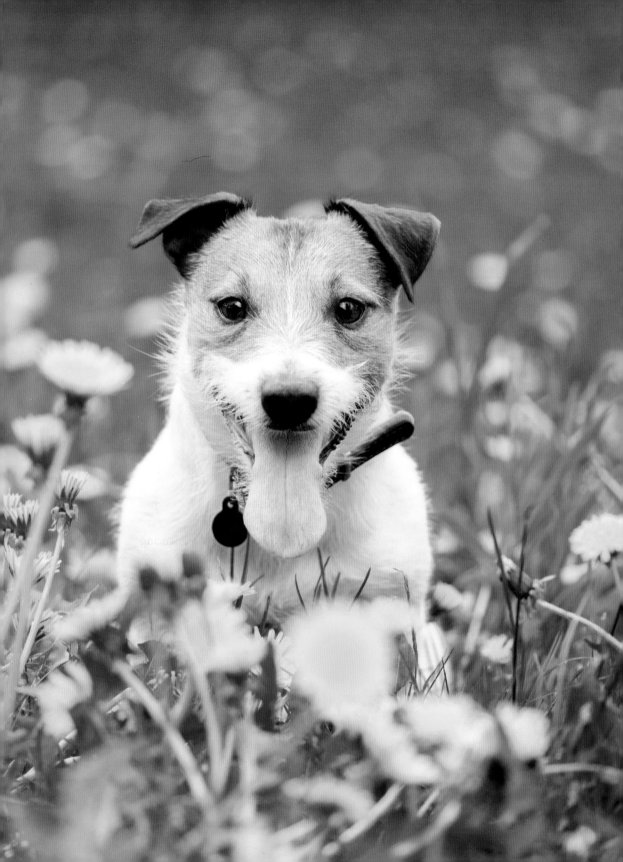

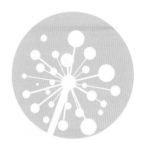

Introduction: Sharing Stories

No one ever watches an itching, chewing, biting, fur-ripping dog or cat and considers it an evening of inexpensive family entertainment. No kid says, "Hey, Mom! Look at the dog! Isn't he funny?" Instead, the family members feel their pet's discomfort: "Stop itching! Please, stop!"

Diarrhea isn't a pleasant diversion, either. Accidents in the house, constant concern over a pet's diet, and frequent visits to the veterinarian aren't really among the good things in life. The incidence of IBD (irritable bowel disease) in cats has been rapidly escalating for years and has just about reached epidemic proportions. Numerous companies, over the years, have formulated special foods for cats experiencing chronic and sometimes debilitating diarrhea.

Pruritis (itching of the skin) and intestinal disorders, such as IBD, have become so very prevalent that it's seriously alarming. In my opinion, our relationship with our pets is supposed to enhance our lives while we enhance theirs. In four decades of veterinary practice, I've grown to understand that both *obtaining* health and *maintaining* health in our pets do not have to be constant struggles.

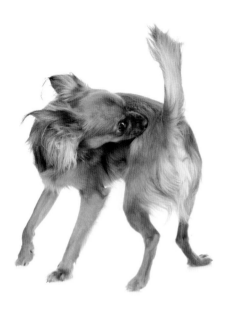

Regarding problems with diet, food allergies are not the same as food sensitivities (or intolerances). Food sensitivities are much more common than food allergies, but food allergies are a real problem, too.

A person with an allergic pet typically follows a path of avoidance. Pet owners will carefully read labels to circumvent foods to which their pets are allergic. However, allergy patients will often subsequently become allergic to ingredients in new foods if they eat them day after day. For example, a pet that was never allergic to lamb may become allergic to lamb because of repeated exposure to it.

Older drugs, like Benadryl and steroids, don't work nearly as well anymore. Therefore, veterinarians often prescribe new drugs, which often handle the itching, routinely. But using these drugs is a catch-22 because they impair very necessary vital functions in the animals' bodies.

It doesn't have to be this way. If you've been dealing with allergies for years with your own pet, it may be hard for you to believe that you can cure allergies. In this book, you're going to learn how to find out what is wrong with your dog or cat. You're also going to learn what you can do about it.

I've written this book to help you cure your pets of allergies and food sensitivities and intolerances. You don't have to spend your life running to the veterinarian over and over again, having your pets allergy-tested, and reading ingredient lists. You don't have to give medications that alter your pet's immune-system function. (Our pets, now more than ever, need good immune systems because cancer is so very prevalent.) It's just as important to know how to prevent allergies and how to start your puppy or kitten off on the right track. Let's look at some stories of allergic pets and their diagnoses and paths to wellness.

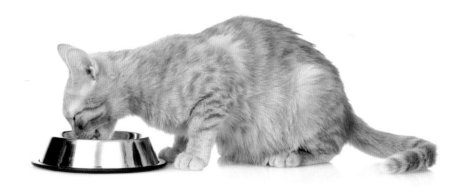

Nellie's Story

Nellie's allergies began shortly after her first birthday. The typical regime of steroids and antibiotics helped only while she was taking them. When her mom tried to cut back on the medications, Nellie's itching and scratching returned with a vengeance. In those days, certain newer (and what I consider even more dangerous) drugs were not available.

I tested Nellie using my Allergy Elimination 4 Pets technique and then used this procedure to reprogram her system so she would no longer experience allergic reactions to the identified foods and environmental triggers. She began to improve after the first visit. "As the treatments progressed, she scratched less and less, the hair under her neck and on her paws grew back, and her skin returned to normal," says Nellie's mom. "After a few months, she stopped scratching altogether. Her coat is now soft and bright, and she feels like a brand-new dog!"

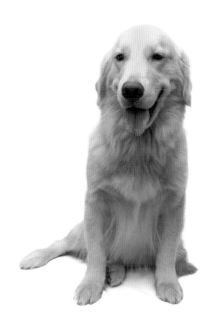

Truman's Story, Told by His Owner

Truman is a Bouvier des Flandres. He was six years old when we began Dr. Khalsa's Allergy Elimination 4 Pets technique. We brought Truman home as a puppy in October 2008, and in November 2008 he began frantically biting at his rear legs and licking and chewing on his feet. Many times, his feet would be raw from chewing. He had constant ear infections and suffered from terrible gas, accompanied by soft and runny stools. After countless visits to a slew of different veterinarians, the episodes of chewing and gas continued.

We tried different foods, including grain-free and limited-ingredient diets, with no improvement. Before I went to Dr. Khalsa, another veterinarian treated him and changed

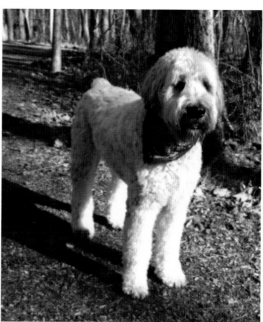

Truman is now a healthy dog with no allergic symptoms.

his diet to all-beef raw. I gave the raw diet for more than two months, but the stool problems, gas, and itching remained.

Many years ago, when Dr. Khalsa had her practice in Yardley, Pennsylvania, she was my veterinarian for many of my cats and dogs. I would drive an hour and a half each way because the drive was worth it to have her treat my pet kids. In April of 2014, I reached out to Dr. Khalsa again and scheduled a phone consult with her to discuss Truman's itching, chewing, and gas. We discussed her Allergy Elimination 4 Pets technique, and I decided to go with it. The great part was that I could do it all at home.

After the Allergy Elimination treatment, I slowly started introducing different foods into Truman's diet. Finally, more than six years after we brought Truman into our life, he is itch-free, he no longer chews his feet, and he has no more horrible episodes of gas. He eats a raw diet with protein sources other than strictly beef. I add vegetables and garlic to his diet, and I give him Deserving Pets Canine Everyday Essentials supplements.

Many veterinarians prescribe drugs that mask the symptoms rather than cure the ailment. After years of Truman's suffering, going to numerous veterinarians, and having him tested, all it took was a phone consultation with Dr. Khalsa to find the treatment that finally gave Truman the relief I had sought for years. Dr. Khalsa offered a drug-free approach to freeing Truman of his allergies.

Goose's Story, Told by His Owner

Goose, our gray cat with green eyes, started plucking tufts of hair from his back around the age of one. At first, it was occasional and hardly even noticeable. As the problem escalated, I would come home from work to find piles of hair in all of his usual hangouts.

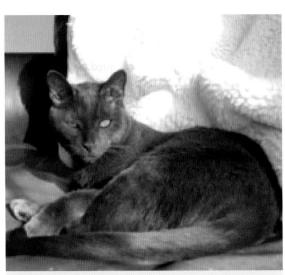
Goose's gray coat is now healthy, full, and shiny.

To watch him do it was painful. He would attack his back and rip the hair in frenetic bursts. My cat was self-mutilating.

I made an appointment with my regular veterinarian. She did blood tests, fungus tests, bacteria tests, parasite tests, even IQ tests (just kidding)—all were inconclusive. My vet's best guess was food allergies.

We started trying different prescription limited-ingredient diets. We had three cats at the time, and there was always one of them who didn't like the food. Separate feedings were nightmarish.

Weeks would pass, and it would seem as if the plucking was subsiding. Maybe

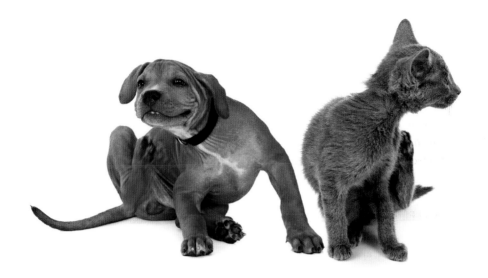

the food was working? Some hair would start to grow back, and then, suddenly, the telltale piles would appear again, often accompanied by bouts of diarrhea and almost daily vomiting.

Goose was scrawny, usually weighing around 7 pounds, and the 2×4-inch bald patch on his back was beyond unsightly. This ebb-and-flow cycle continued for more than two years.

We concluded that Goose's allergies were partly food-related and partly seasonal. We would control what we could with diet and then medicate through the bad stretches. I knew he didn't feel well, but I was helpless and certain that we had exhausted our options.

Then I found Dr. Khalsa and had a consult. She did Allergy Elimination 4 Pets with Goose. My husband, who wasn't into holistic practices, had a field day with my journey into the world of holistic veterinary medicine. He delighted in telling friends and family that I had invented new and unusual ways to spend money on our cat.

As we did the treatments (totally noninvasive, by the way), my husband adopted the same look each night: part resignation and part disgust. Our friends were in stitches over the stories of these holistic treatments, and I played along, figuring that, at the very least, I had bought a great way to entertain others.

But then…

Before we knew it, months had passed without Goose plucking one hair. I thought maybe it was just an unusually long good stretch, and surely it was only a matter of time before I would happen upon a nest of plucked hair and feel the wave of dread wash over me (I can be pretty dramatic). But there was no denying it: this was out of the ordinary. Not only had Goose's hair grown in, but he was filling out, had stopped vomiting, and was playing like a kitten.

I was so afraid of a relapse that I said nothing, figuratively holding my breath with hope. When Goose had his regular check-up, he had gained more than a pound. Really? My mother, who affectionately referred to Goose as "Rat" because of his pathetic appearance, remarked, "That's not

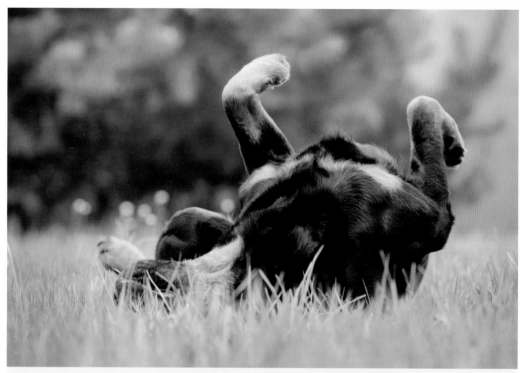

A roll in the grass can cause itchiness and other problems for an allergic pet.

the same cat." I welled up when a friend, fishing for the latest comedic update, inquired, "How's kitty's treatment going?" and my husband answered, "I think it worked."

Maddie's Story, Told by Her Owner

At our first appointment with Dr. Khalsa, we read some testimonials and prayed that someday we could also write one. I had been brainwashed to believe that traditional medicine was the best and only way to treat our four-year-old English Bulldog, Maddie. The nightmare had started in July 2000, when 44-pound Maddie developed an extreme case of diarrhea. Every time we stopped the medication that our veterinarian gave us, her stools became liquid. Her weight plummeted to 35 pounds in three weeks. Blood tests showed elevated pancreatic and liver enzymes with the albumen and total protein in her blood dropping. Our regular vet recommended that we see a gastrointestinal specialist, so we made an appointment immediately.

Maddie was diagnosed with an extreme case of IBD and a small liver, which could complicate things due to the medication that the vet prescribed: prednisolone, azathioprine, furosemide, metronidazole, and metoclopamide. The specialist told us that this approach was around 70 percent successful and that it would take a month to see results. Two weeks after beginning the medications, she was down to 32 pounds. The fluid in her abdomen worsened, and she was now vomiting.

In late August, Maddie went into convulsions, and we drove her to a renowned veterinary hospital in our area. After three days there, she was rediagnosed with the same problems plus lymphangiectasia, a condition in which the GI tract loses its ability to absorb nutrients. Four weeks of treatment in intensive care and $14,000 later, the vets recommended that we put Maddie to sleep. She now weighed 25 pounds and was just skin and bone. We took her home and kept her alive with calcium injections and special intravenous feedings that would increase the protein in her blood.

In mid-October, Maddie had her first appointment with Dr. Khalsa and began Allergy Elimination 4 Pets treatments. After the first treatment, Maddie's condition remained stable, and on some days she had semiformed stools and some energy. Her leaky gut also began to stabilize. After just two treatments, we were able to stop the calcium injections and special IV feedings. Her blood-test results started moving toward normal. By January 2001, Maddie no longer needed any medications. She weighed 36 pounds and was jumping on the sofa and playing like she used to.

(Dr. Khalsa's note: Maddie went on to live a normal, long life, and she died at a ripe old age for an English Bulldog.)

The Path to Relief

Owners of allergic pets: I've created this book just for you—to fully educate you about allergies and sensitivities. We'll talk about how to prevent them, how to treat them, and why they're so awfully common in today's world. I've included separate sections on skin problems and gastrointestinal problems. I hope, someday, because of this book, you can have a success story like Nellie's, Truman's, Goose's, or Maddie's.

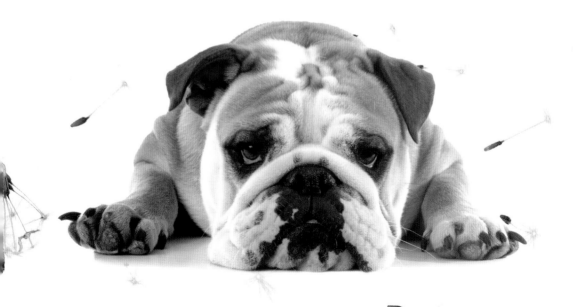

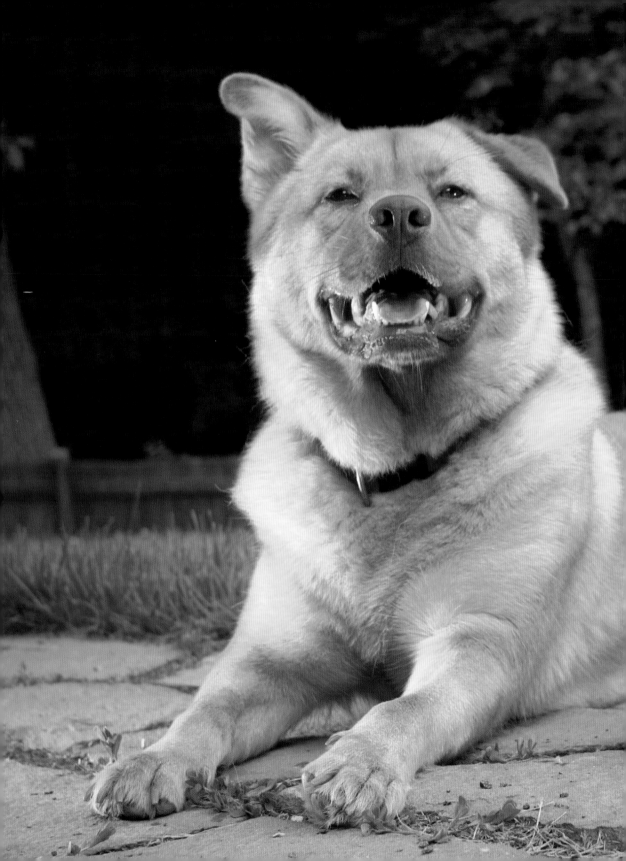

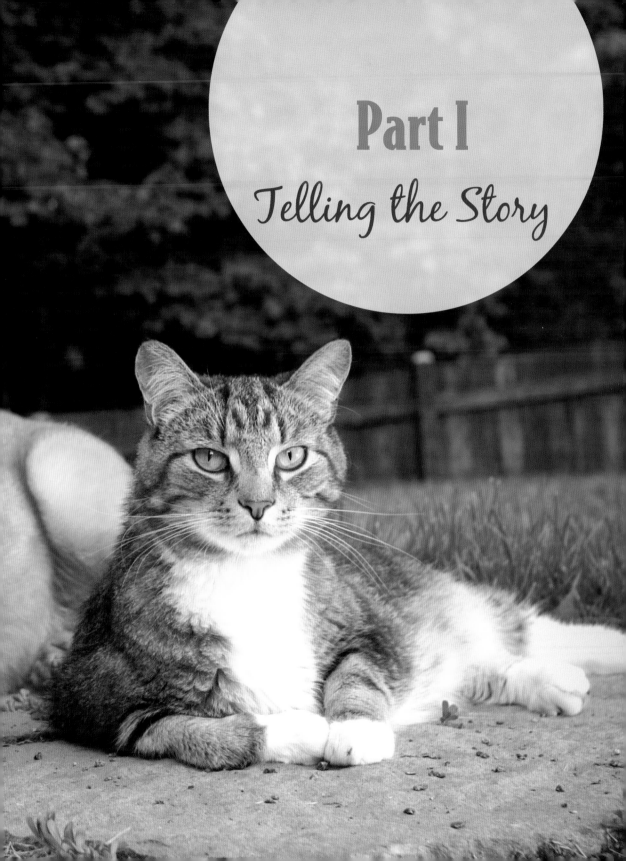

Part I
Telling the Story

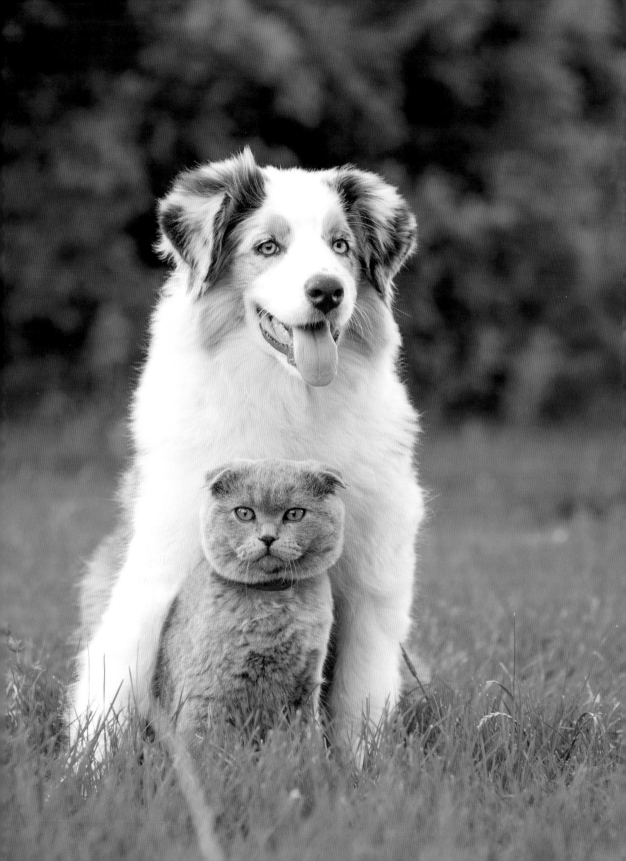

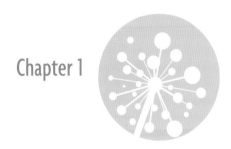

Chapter 1

Holistic Health:
Understanding Your Pet's Body

Holistic health is all about keeping your pet as healthy as he or she can be. Your pet's body is a complex machine, bustling with activity and full of energy. How well this machine is maintained will define how healthy your pet will remain and how long his or her life will be.

Allergies drain energy away from your pet's important bodily functions. Allergies also work to exhaust your pet's immune system. That's why handling allergies until you completely eliminate them is so important in providing your pet with a healthy and long life. Preventing allergies is just as, if not more, important.

Conventional therapies tend to "take over" and corrupt the natural healing function of the body, actually decreasing the body's ability to heal itself. Likewise, stopping conventional therapies, such as corticosteroids, just about always results in the problem remaining just as bad or getting even worse. Pets can become dependent upon medications that are not good for them.

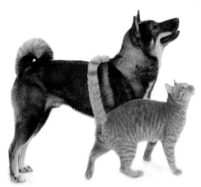
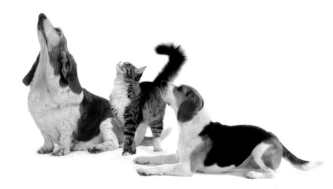

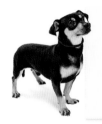
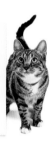

Our pets' bodies have systems that keep them healthy and work to prevent disease. Certain conventional medications disrupt these systems in order to alleviate the allergic symptoms. And, in fact, *alleviate* is all that they do—they don't in any way, shape, or form cure allergies. It's important to know that these medications alleviate symptoms by impeding important protective functions that keep our pets safe from other diseases, including cancer. I discuss this in more detail later in the book. In modern times, when one out of two dogs will get cancer, we want our pet's immune systems in tip-top shape.

All of the holistic procedures that you are going to learn about are important developments in the history of healing. Many of them work to correct problems and some work to fully eliminate problems. These holistic techniques work with the body to fortify and encourage its own healing powers. The end result is a healthier patient with a stronger immune system.

Today, terms like *conventional*, *holistic*, *alternative*, and *complementary* abound in medical literature. These words are used so often and in so many contexts that one begins to wonder what these terms really mean.

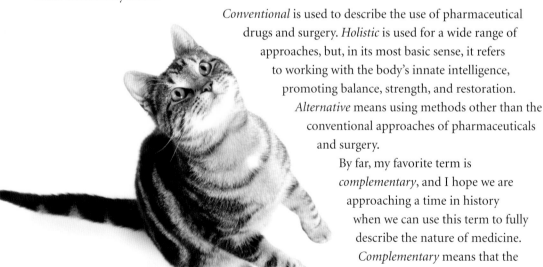

Conventional is used to describe the use of pharmaceutical drugs and surgery. *Holistic* is used for a wide range of approaches, but, in its most basic sense, it refers to working with the body's innate intelligence, promoting balance, strength, and restoration. *Alternative* means using methods other than the conventional approaches of pharmaceuticals and surgery.

By far, my favorite term is *complementary*, and I hope we are approaching a time in history when we can use this term to fully describe the nature of medicine. *Complementary* means that the wonderful medley of healing styles, both new and ancient, can be

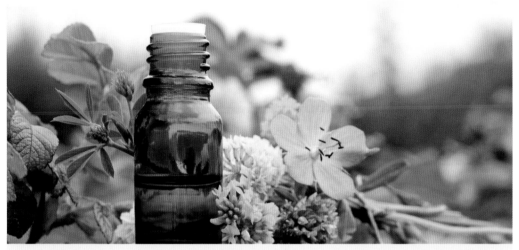

Homeopathic and herbal remedies may be part of a holistic treatment plan.

used to complement each other. There is a time and a place for each and every one. The ability to combine the best options from different healing approaches is what's known as integrative health care and complementary medicine.

This book discusses integrative health care to give you many options for healing your pet along with a full understanding of the subject. When we give our dogs' and cats' systems the ammunition they need to run properly and the guidance they need to correct disease-causing problems, our pets can rapidly heal. All holistic modalities/techniques have the same common denominator in that they greatly increase the body's ability to heal and cure itself. It's that simple.

The body's cells are always working at a furious pace toward order and health. They are well acquainted with the actions necessary to continue in their pursuit of life. Holistic therapies only help them in their endeavor.

Holistic care contains therapies that make up powerfully healing combinations. In learning about some simple holistic health therapies for allergies and skin problems, you'll be able care for many of your pet's needs. You'll have to read this book carefully, but you'll reap the rewards once you understand the basics and apply them.

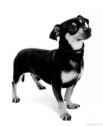

Did You Know?

Holistic health works with the nature of healing because there's a perfect innate wisdom that's always at work.

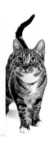

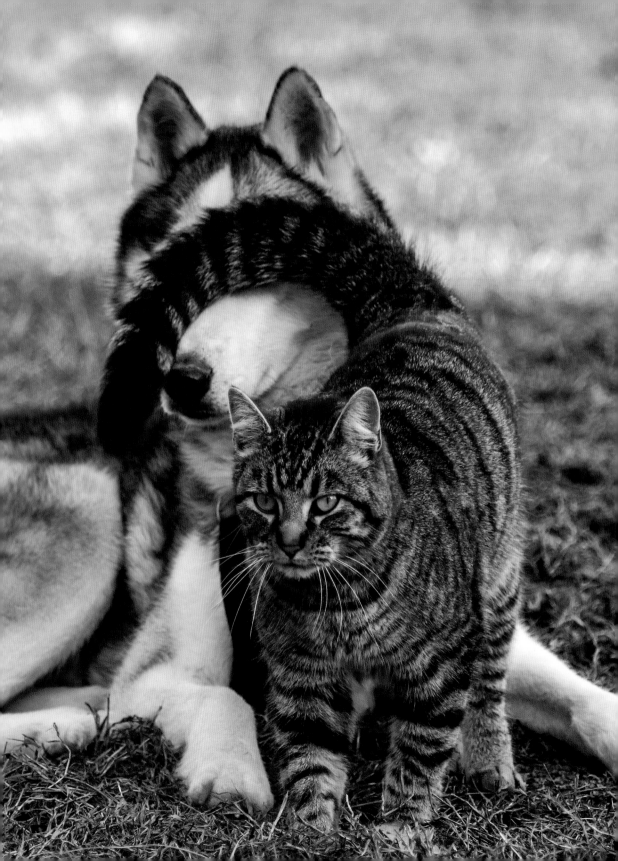

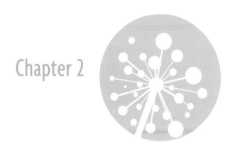

Chapter 2

The Story of Allergies: The Misbehaving Immune System

Ａll pet allergies have a common denominator: an animal who has lost the ability to cope with his or her environment. The best way to understand allergies is to understand how the immune system works.

Let me compare the immune system to a computer. Much like how a computer processes and recalls data, an immune system will identify and remember various enemies. That's why if we get measles once, we won't ever get this illness again—the immune system sees the measles germs trying to get a foot in the door, recognizes them as an enemy, and slams the door in their face. The immune system remembers the measles from the previous infection and handles the problem immediately.

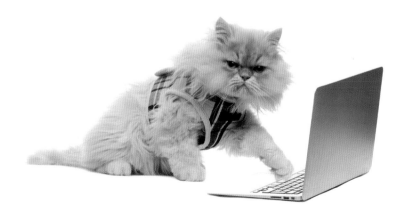

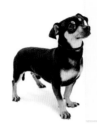

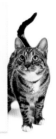

In the case of allergies, the immune system incorrectly processes and registers "good guys" as enemies. Foods, pollens, and grasses, among others, are identified by the body as threats (allergens). These threats warrant responses, and the subsequent responses cause inflammation and other allergic symptoms. The immune system becomes a virus-corrupted computer.

Consider the young child who has a severe reaction to peanuts. His friend can eat a peanut butter sandwich without any ill effects. That's because the computer of his friend's immune systems hasn't logged the peanut in as an enemy. The problem isn't the peanut itself. Rather, it's the way that the immune system recognizes the peanut.

Today's pets are experiencing more allergies because there are simply more ways to confuse their immune systems. Nature never designed our pets' systems to be exposed to so many vaccinations, chemicals and pesticides on a routine basis. A confused immune system results in an increased number of items that are logged in as enemies.

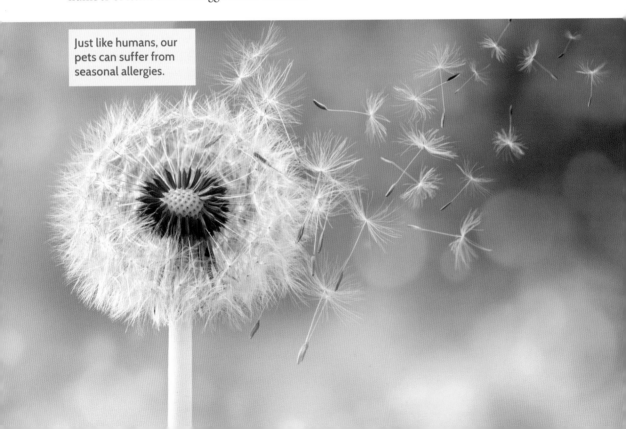

Just like humans, our pets can suffer from seasonal allergies.

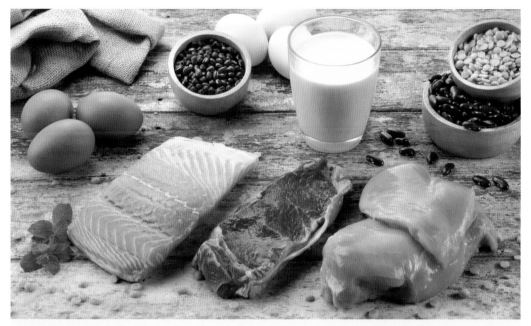

Changing your pet's protein source may, but doesn't always, help ease allergic symptoms.

All of these incorrectly logged-in enemies—allergens—can individually cause an allergic reaction in our pet's body, and each individual item adds to the allergic burden. Most allergic dogs and cats are allergic to numerous things. But, simply eating the problematic foods may not be enough in itself to get their immune systems aggravated to the point where itching or diarrhea occurs. However, when even more allergens, such as additional food triggers or environmental allergens (e.g., seasonal pollens and molds) are added to the mix, the total number of allergens present will reach high enough concentrations to bring on those allergic symptoms, such as chronic itching. The foods play a big part in the overall allergic reaction, while the pollens are the straw that broke the camel's back.

Another example is a cat who is very sensitive to fish and less sensitive to beef. The sum of the whole occurs when a tiny bit of fish used for flavoring the food along with the beef causes an allergic response, resulting in chronic diarrhea. Because when enough allergens are present, they will exceed the body's threshold.

When the immune system is busy dealing with unnecessary reactions to food and environmental allergens, it is not present to fight bacterial infections, cancer, and other insults to the body and vital force. Releasing the immune system from the burden of allergies brings about a dramatic increase in energy, health, and well-being. Imagine yourself running around and putting out fires in your neighbors' homes and then realizing too late that your own house is on fire. Aside from diverting the body and immune system from the important work they need to do, allergies exhaust the body's *qi* (life force), cause imbalances and disharmony, and cause the body to retain toxins.

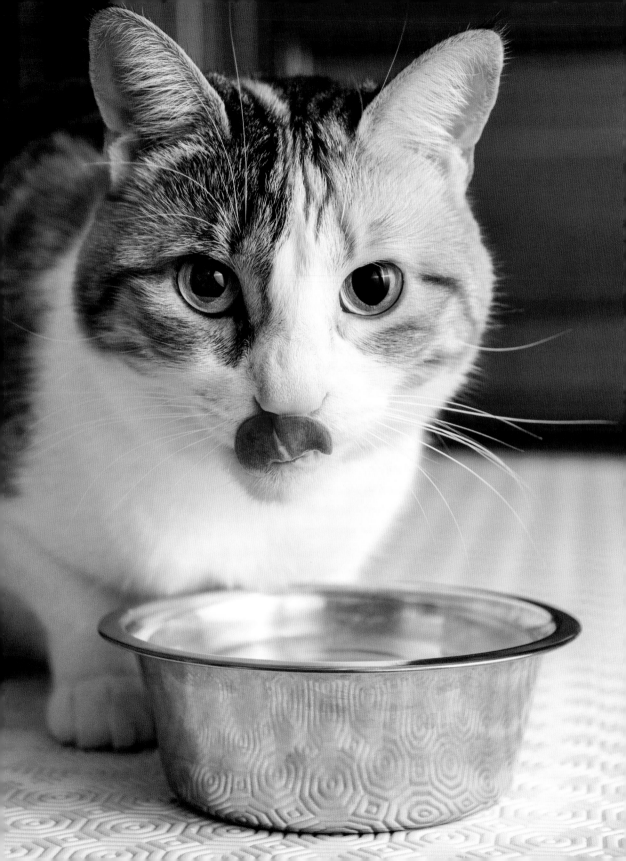

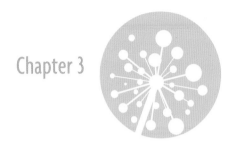

Chapter 3

The Phenolic Component: Food Sensitivities and More

Food Sensitivities/Intolerances

Food allergies and food sensitivities, or intolerances, are not the same thing. The talk of the town is always about food *allergies*, yet food *sensitivities* (also called food *intolerances*) are fifteen times more common than food allergies. Pet owners and veterinarians alike have tended to bunch them all into one category: "allergies." But that's not what's actually happening. Because allergies and sensitivities are not well understood, dog owners run to switch from food to food, wondering why radical diet changes aren't working.

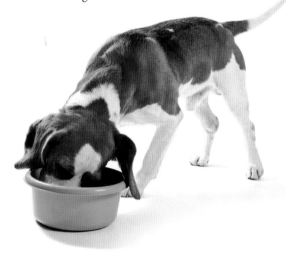

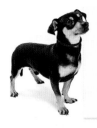

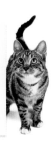

Did You Know?

The reaction in the gut becomes a battle that can easily escalate to wild bouts of itching, diarrhea, gas, and irritable bowel syndrome.

We've also got to differentiate between food-related problems and environmental allergies, sensitivities, and intolerances. Understanding the difference will help you figure out and handle what's really going on in a pet with an itching or GI problem. Let's discuss the differences between an allergy and an intolerance.

With a bona fide food allergy, your pet's body produces antibodies called immunoglobulins, specifically immunoglobulin E (IgE) and immunoglobulin G (IgG). They can cause itching, hives, rashes, sudden diarrhea, or a combination of any of these. Environmental allergens, when inhaled, may also prompt your pet's immune system to produce these specific antibodies. In all cases, mast cells become activated and begin to produce *histamine*, which causes a rapid inflammatory response. A true allergy produces an immediate response. Consider the kid with peanut allergies or asthma attacks.

Food intolerances, or sensitivities, create a delayed immune response. Different antibodies, called immunoglobulin A (IgA) and immunoglobulin M (IgM), live in the walls of the intestine. It's important to know that food intolerances cause a delayed response in the intestine. In other words, your dog can eat the offending food on Monday, and the reaction can occur much later in the week or even later in the month. That makes pinning down the culprit a difficult task. Food intolerances will also build up over time because our dogs eat the same thing over and over again; this repetition helps create food intolerances.

It's pretty typical for a dog parent to sigh in relief, if not jump for joy, when he or she finally finds a food that agrees with a dog with IBD. Unfortunately, the owner then feeds that food day after day, greatly increasing the chance that the dog will later develop a reaction to the new food. Because

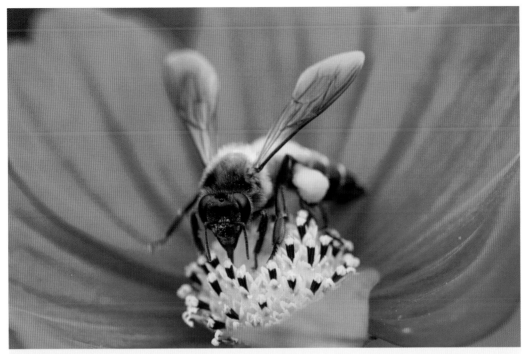

Environmental allergens can combine with food-related issues to make your pet miserable.

it often takes time and repeated exposure for food intolerances and sensitivities to manifest, I firmly believe that it's important to feed a rotating diet.

There have been some important breakthroughs in the treatment of food sensitivities. In the late 1970s, Robert Gardner, PhD, a professor of animal science at Brigham Young University in Provo, Utah, discovered agents called *phenolics* that can cause immune reactions. Phenolics are regularly found throughout our environment. These compounds are naturally present in foods. In fact, they're responsible for a food's taste and smell. Phenolic compounds color, flavor, and

Did You Know?

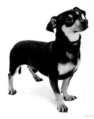

There's a lot of confusion about switching from diet to diet. In many cases, switching to a completely different protein doesn't improve the pet's condition. The problem lies in the fact that phenolic compounds are everywhere and in just about everything.

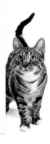

preserve foods. They protect plants against pathogens, help in the dispersal and germination of seeds, and attract flower pollinators. A flower might have bee-attracting phenolics, while a carrot may have insect-repelling phenolics to protect it from being eaten.

While phenolic compounds naturally occur in all foods, they may also be found in pollens, chemicals, and other nonfood substances. They're tiny molecules that have the ability to stimulate the immune system. They tend to cause delayed reactions, which can affect any tissue in the body.

Phenolics aren't easy to avoid. In fact, I can say with confidence that they're impossible to avoid. One food alone can contain several phenolics, while one single phenolic can be in hundreds of different foods.

One particular phenolic, gallic acid, is the culprit in many cases of food sensitivity. It's present in 70 percent of foods, including almonds, avocado, banana, barley, beef, beets, blueberry, cabbage, chicken, corn, cow's milk, duck, eggs, honey, lamb, millet, oats, peas, pumpkin, raspberry, rice, soy, squash, turkey, wheat bran, yams, and yeast (again, these are just *some* of the common foods that contain gallic acid). So, if your dog is sensitive to gallic acid, he could have an adverse reaction to any or all of these foods.

As I mentioned previously, while one single phenolic, such as gallic acid, can be present in hundreds of different foods, most foods actually contain multiple phenolics. As just one example, wheat contains coumarin, gallic acid, quercetin, and rutin. These particular phenolics all commonly cause food intolerances. In contrast, rabbit works very well in dogs and cats with

Switching Foods

You do an allergy test and find out that your dog is reacting to beef, chicken, sweet potato, corn, and soy. You go off to the store, carrying a magnifying glass so you can read all of the ingredient lists on the food packages. You proudly choose a food with duck, or maybe lamb, as the protein, and it's also made with peas. Sound perfect? Well, if you look at the foregoing list, everything you chose also contains gallic acid. If your dog is sensitive to this phenolic, you will have little success with this diet change. So if you've been switching from food to food, changing brands and protein sources and ingredients, you can now see why it can be very difficult to find a food that "works" for your pet.

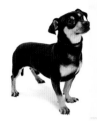

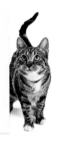

chronic GI problems because, besides being a novel protein, it contains one rather innocent phenolic called piperine.

Doctors have been using homeopathic phenolic neutralization and desensitization techniques to help people overcome their sensitivities. The same can be done for pets. The use of a simple oral remedy to treating symptoms is a very effective method to help reduce food and environmental intolerances and sensitivities. It's equivalent to a homeopathic remedy.

Deseret Biologicals makes a gallic acid desensitizing phenolic compound that you can give orally to your pet. They also offer similar compounds for other phenolics individually. In my consulting practice, I often use a phenolic desensitizing combination that includes multiple phenolic compounds in homeopathic form so I can eliminate the reaction to a number of those pesky phenolics during one course of treatment.

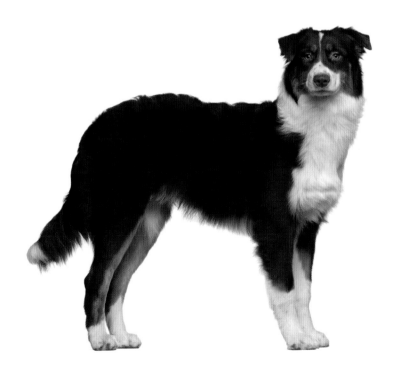

Perhaps now it's easier to understand why changing ingredients in your dog's food didn't work as well as you anticipated. Without Dr. Gardner's important work and findings regarding phenolics, we'd be without any cure for this all-too-common problem in our pets.

Phenolics and Feline Asthma

Asthma in cats is very similar to asthma in humans. Both are the result of chronic inflammation of the small passageways of the lungs. When these passageways constrict, it makes it very difficult for the person or cat to breathe.

The signs of asthma include a persistent cough and wheezing. Some cats with milder cases of asthma get only a very slight but chronic cough. In more advanced cases, a cat will squat, with his shoulders hunched and his neck extended, experiencing rapid breathing or even gasping for breath. Cats with asthma can also have open-mouth breathing and can gag up foamy mucus.

Asthma is an allergic bronchitis that is set in motion when the lungs become inflamed in reaction to a substance. If your cat shows asthma symptoms, your veterinarian will likely take a

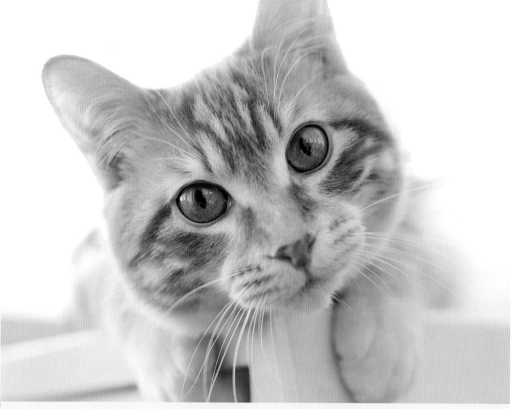

Knowledge about phenolics can help you keep your cat breathing freely.

Phenolics that Affect Asthmatics

Coumarin: Found in at least thirty foods, including wheat, rice, barley, corn, soy, cheese, beef, lamb, pumpkin, yam, yeast, and eggs.

Indole: This compound represents the amino acid tryptophan, which can be transformed by bacteria into indole. It is in all complete proteins and has been found to aggravate asthma.

Malvin: Found in approximately thirty-five foods, including chicken, eggs, milk, soy, and corn, malvin is second only to gallic acid in its allergic response and is associated with asthma.

Note: Although gallic acid is a major instigator of food-related problems, it is not implicated in asthma.

chest x-ray to rule out any other possible problems that can cause similar symptoms, such as a heart condition. Often, there are telltale signs on the chest x-ray that will indicate asthma.

Conventional advice is to avoid using perfumes, room fresheners, carpet deodorizers, aerosol cleaners, and the like around cats with asthma. The reason for this is not commonly known: asthma is typically caused by allergic reactions from both airborne phenolic compounds and phenolics found in foods. Airborne phenolic compounds are often found in pollen, tobacco smoke, house dust, air pollution, kapok (a cotton-like fiber from the tree of the same name), wool, feathers, animal hair or dander, building materials, furniture stuffing, cottonseed, and chemical odors. They're ubiquitous and particularly present in the products we use around the house; the compounds that create fragrance are, typically, phenolics.

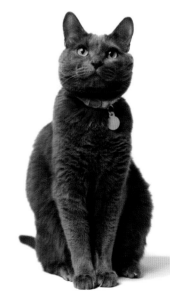

Although the research about the relationship between asthma and phenolics has been done with humans, I feel it is applicable to our feline friends, too. The thing is, nowadays we're all exposed to phenolics almost everywhere. The good news is that cats can be treated to become desensitized to phenolics by administering the compounds orally as liquid homeopathic remedies; coumarin and indole are the two most important phenolics in regard to asthma. Additonally, the homeopathic products AllerCyl AirBorn and AllerCyl Breathe also work to desensitize your cat to these two common phenolics.

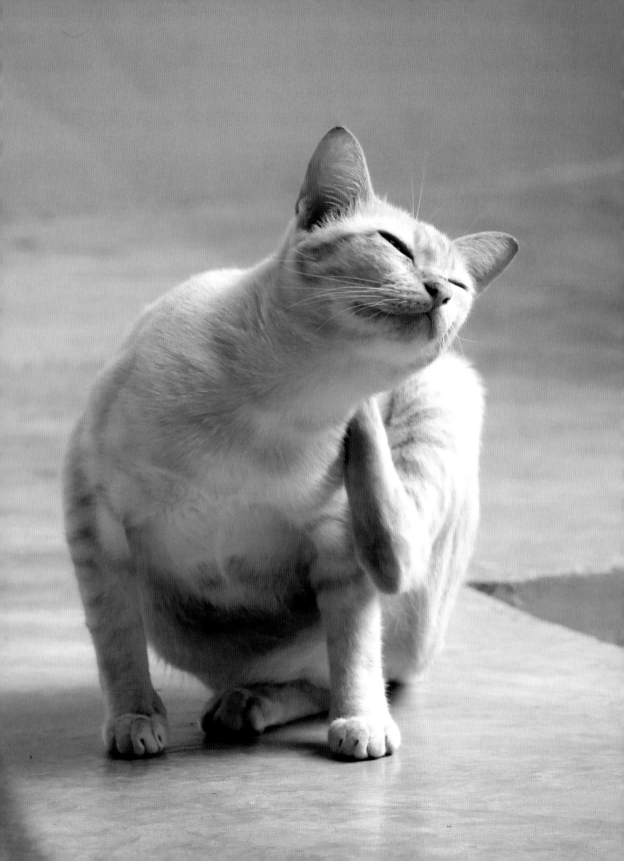

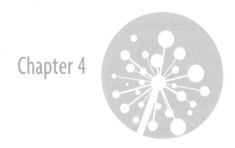

Chapter 4

An Epidemic of Itching: Why Allergies Have Become Very Common

As far as allergic itching goes, there's a difference between our pets' reaction to allergens and our human reaction. That's because dogs and cats have the inflammatory cells that react to allergens all over their bodies, while humans have them mostly in the respiratory tract. If we were set up for allergies like our pets, we'd be scratching our rumps and chewing on our arms during ragweed season!

When an allergen is inhaled, ingested, or contacted, it causes the immune system to produce special proteins: immunoglobulin E and immunoglobulin G (IgE and IgG). These immunoglobulin proteins attach to cells called *mast cells*.

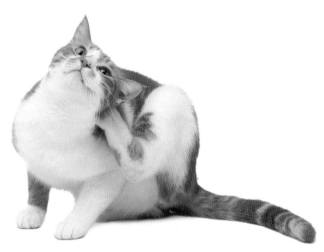

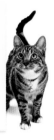

Did You Know?

Allergies can result in itching, skin infections, hot spots, ear infections, frequent or chronic diarrhea, vomiting, seizures, behavior problems, pancreatitis, hyperactivity, chronic liver disease, lethargy, and even cancer.

The mast cells then release histamine and other inflammatory chemicals, which cause all of that itching and irritation.

The histamine has an "open-sesame" effect on the capillaries, causing redness and inflammation. Dogs have ten times the amount of mast cells in their skin that humans do, and these mast cells are located all over their bodies. Cats have an abundance of mast cells in their skin, too. That's why our dogs and cats wind up chewing at many different areas on their bodies when they're allergic to something.

I've found that food allergies form the important base of the pyramid with all of the environmental allergens piled on top. When a dog comes to my practice itching ferociously from fleas, I know that the flea is not the sole cause of the problem. The flea sits on the top of the pyramid and is the straw that breaks the camel's back.

The age of onset of an allergic condition can depend on inheritance. The stronger the genetic factor that predisposes a pet to allergies, the earlier the onset can be. The tendency toward an

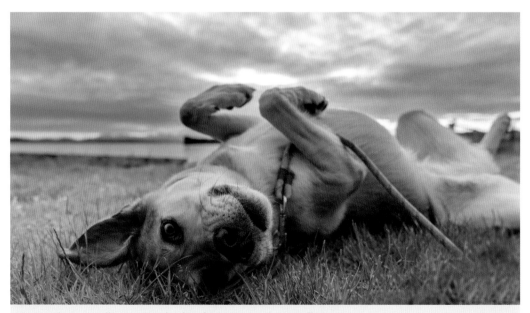

Your pet's mast cells go to work when he is exposed to an allergen.

allergic disposition is likely inherited. Yet, sensitivity to any specific allergen is not inherited. That said, pets' exposure to poisons, toxins, and multiple vaccinations is certainly a game-changer. When your dog's or cat's body becomes stressed or imbalanced, allergic symptoms begin to appear, and the body's defenses become overworked and exhausted.

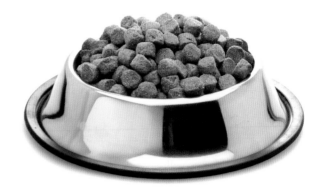

An allergy can be defined as a "hypersensitive state acquired through exposure to a particular allergen." Repeated exposure is an important part of the development of an allergy. Doctors often become allergic to latex because they put on and take off latex examination gloves many times each day, so they then must start using latex-free gloves. If doctors didn't use latex gloves so frequently on a daily basis, they would be much less likely to develop an allergy to latex.

Let's look at the example of a pet who is allergic to chicken and beef but switches to a lamb diet and does very well. Therefore, the pet stays on the lamb-based diet every day, without variation. Based on my experience, I'd predict that this pet would become allergic to lamb within six months. Likewise, many cats are allergic to fish because it's found so abundantly in cat food because cats like the flavor.

Why is it that so many of our pets' internal computer programs are going haywire? One likely explanation is that multiple vaccinations (many of them unnecessary) have worked to confuse their immune systems, causing an exaggerated response. Their immune systems were never designed to ward off simultaneous incursions by several different agents. Looking at it in human context, I know of no recorded cases in which a person was exposed to polio, smallpox, measles, mumps, and whooping cough all at one time.

The immune system's design is compatible with the laws of statistics, meaning that it just isn't set up to handle such a multipronged attack because the chance of its occurrence is just so low. But such an attack on the immune system is exactly what multivalent combination vaccinations simulate. The immune system is being asked to recognize and fight off, all at once, all of the vaccine components. For a dog, this means distemper, parvovirus, leptospirosis, adenovirus, hepatitis, and bordetella, and perhaps also coronavirus, rabies, and Lyme disease. For a cat, this means feline distemper, panleukopenia, viral rhinotracheitis, coronavirus, rabies, and FeLV (feline leukemia virus). In addition to antigens and viruses, vaccinations contain formaldehyde and mercury. Neither our dogs' nor our cats' immune systems were designed to have multiple disease organisms, antigens, and toxic substances injected into the body at one time, as is the case with vaccines.

Even more significant in these vaccines are the tiny bits of chicken and cow material left over from the chicken embryo and bovine serum in which the viruses are incubated. Unfortunately, when these food products are introduced to the body with the other invaders, that's how the body's internal computer is likely to identify them. Just imagine yourself living in a house on the prairie and being attacked by a gang of a dozen outlaws. As you prepare to defend yourself from the invaders, would you try to differentiate between them to decide if perhaps some were benign? Or would you register them all as enemies? You'd likely do the latter, and that's exactly what the immune system is prone to do.

It's actually no coincidence that the first foods usually removed from an allergic pet's diet are chicken and beef, kissing cousins to the egg and bovine serum used to incubate vaccine viruses. The pet is then likely switched to a "hypoallergenic diet," typically consisting of lamb and rice. But the proteins in lamb are not so far removed from those in beef, and because the dog or cat is usually fed the same thing every day, he or she will soon become allergic to lamb, too.

The concerned owner may switch to wild game, such as venison or rabbit, but these foods, too, soon begin to trigger the animal's immune system to put up a fight. After going through a veritable dietary petting zoo, the hypoallergenic food of last resort is a special predigested protein. So palliating the problem by changing the food tends to be only a short-term fix at best.

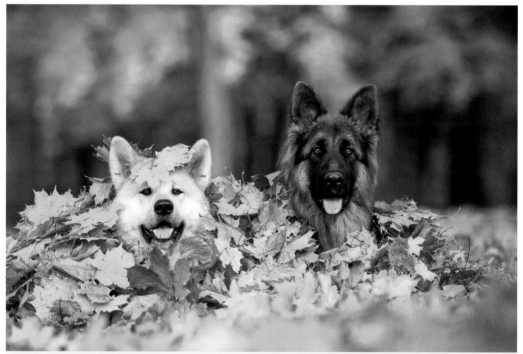

Seasonal allergy triggers are not limited to springtime.

Another factor that influences the occurrence of allergic reactions is seasonal change. In northern climes, the coming of winter, when grass, weeds, trees, and pollen become dormant and covered over, some allergy-prone animals may experience some relief; however, others may actually suffer an increase in allergic reactions to dust, molds, and debris from heating systems. In addition, romping in fallen leaves increases a dog's exposure to such potential allergens as fungus, mold, and mildew.

Every season has its own allergy triggers, which affect different pets in different ways. Whereas an allergy trigger might cause us our eyes to itch and water, the same trigger is more likely to irritate the area above a dog's tail, along with other areas of his or her body.

A dog or cat afflicted with skin allergies may develop itching anywhere from the head to the tail—remember, animals have more mast cells than humans do, and these mast cells release histamines in response to certain triggers, causing itching over a pet's entire body. Cats tend to itch and scratch around their ears and faces and lick (often denuding the areas) their stomachs and inside their thighs in response to food allergies. Cats can also get lesions on their lips that look like sores and are called rodent ulcers. Of course, both cats and dogs can experience diarrhea and digestive problems as allergic responses to food allergies or sensitivities. As far as the itchy skin goes, it's just like what your mother told you about mosquito bites: "The more you scratch, the more you itch."

Just as in humans, an allergy occurs when the pet's immune system mistakenly believes that a specific food or environmental substance is harmful. The immune system responds with antibodies, which trigger a series of dangerous symptoms. When the immune system begins acting like a fire department responding to a bunch of false alarms, it is diverted from its intended task, which is to fight bacterial infections, viruses, cancers, and other alien invaders.

Did You Know?

Atopy, the clinical term for inhalant allergies, can account for a significant number of itching dogs. The thing to remember is that it all adds up. The vast majority of dogs who are allergic to foods also have inhalant allergies. The food allergies may not be enough to push them above threshold, but adding pollens, grasses, trees, and weeds to the mix starts a bout of severe itching.

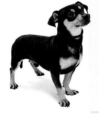

The allergic animal's faulty internal computer will find more and more substances to which to become allergic. As the years pass, the two-week summer allergy becomes a three-month allergy and finally results in year-round problems as your pet's allergies increase.

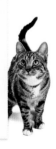

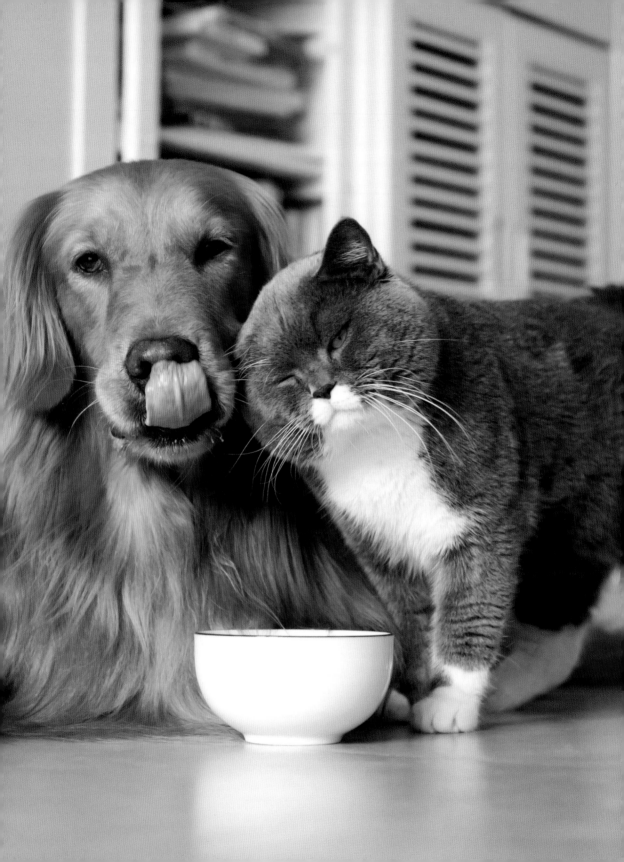

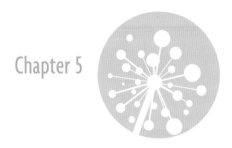

Chapter 5

Battlefield Gut:
The War in Our Pets' Intestines

*I*rritable bowel disease (IBD) is no less than a series of battles going on in the digestive tract of your dog or cat. The body's immune response struggles to defeat the invading armies of foreign substances. The collateral damage suffered from these conflicts results in the symptoms of IBD. The good news is that these clashes and brawls in your pet's gut can be avoided.

Many years ago, as mentioned previously, I heard a lecture by a veterinarian who was highly renowned for his research on IBD. Experience had taught me that questions asked one-on-one were often more candidly answered than those asked in a group setting. That's why I sought out the lecturer afterward and asked him, "Why do you think we're seeing an epidemic rise in IBD?" He replied, "We're vaccinating them with the same stuff we're feeding them." That was in the late 1990s.

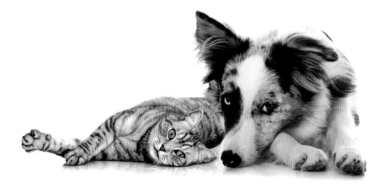

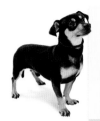
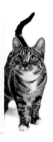

Did You Know?

The intestine does a lot more than simply digest food; in fact, the immune system contains 80 percent of your (and your pet's) immune system.

Why would the components of vaccinations cause IBD? You know from Chapter 4 that vaccines contain chicken embryo and bovine serum. During vaccination, these proteins are introduced into the pet's body along with the other vaccine components. A pet's immune system identifies all of these vaccine components as enemies, and, as far as the immune system is concerned, when any enemy shows its ugly face, it's time for battle. IBD in our pets comes about when the battlefield is in the gut.

Signs of War: Setting Up Camp

With IBD, the soldiers (inflammatory cells) infiltrate the intestinal walls and set up base camp. In the trenches are the regiments, made up of different types of white blood cells, such as lymphocytes, plasmacytes, eosinophils, and sometimes neutrophils. After many battles, the intestinal walls become thickened and cannot absorb nutrients as well as they used to. This collateral damage within the walls of the intestine commonly results in symptoms such as diarrhea, mucus or blood in the stool, vomiting, and weight loss.

Three-Letter Agencies: IgA and IgM

In the US government, three-letter agencies such as the CIA and FBI provide intelligence services and identify enemies. In your pet's body, immunoglobulins (also known as antibodies) are the three-letter agencies that help protect your pet.

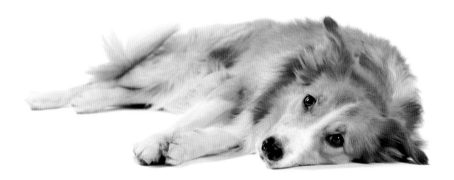

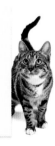

Special immunogloblins, IgA and IgM, live in your pet's digestive tract and serve as the gut's intelligence service by identifying enemies. They initiate the battle in the gut by calling in the regiments: the eosinophils and plasmacytes. This starts the battle of food intolerance, which can easily escalate to all-out war: IBD.

Stealth Invaders: Mycoplasmas

Your dog's body is equipped with a variety of defense mechanisms to help prevent the entrance of perceived intruders, like pathogens, and to destroy them if they do enter the tissues.

But what if that intruder is almost impossible to find? Super-tiny pathogens called *mycoplasmas*—the smallest known microorganisms that self-replicate—elude the immune system. These amorphous little creatures can change their shapes to appear and disappear at will (sort of like jellyfish), concealing themselves within body tissues and body fluids and becoming very difficult to track down.

Because they don't carry any antigenic markers that the immune system can recognize and attack, their presence isn't revealed by blood tests used to detect disease. They can also reemerge from their hiding places inside cells once the coast is clear.

What makes mycoplasmas particularly pernicious is their ability to move into cells and steal the proteins, fats, and vitamins that the cells need to survive (and that they cannot make themselves).

Sometimes described as parasitic bacteria, mycoplasmas have been known to squeeze through filters used to maintain sterility in hospitals and laboratories, and to be sources of contamination in important experiments, routine vaccinations, and more.

To conceal themselves in your pet's body, mycoplasmas use a trick known as *molecular mimicry*—they disguise themselves to resemble the host cells, for instance, by incorporating the cells' surface material into their own jellylike surfaces. This is what may confuse the immune system into attacking the body's own tissues. Your pet's immune system will try to eliminate the mycoplasmas hiding in his GI tract. The immune system will fail to locate the stealth pathogens but, in the attempt, will create inflammatory reactions that cause IBD.

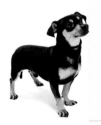

Did You Know?

Food intolerances and sensitivities cause delayed responses in the intestine. In other words, your pet can eat an offending food and not experience a reaction until several days (or even longer) later.

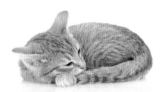

Testing

In both my and Dr. Jean Dodds' opinion, the bottom line with allergic pets is food sensitivities. Conventional tests to determine food allergies, which I consider the base of the pyramid for allergies, are 25 percent accurate. To put it another way, conventional tests for food allergies are 75 percent inaccurate, which means that the resulting "allergic food" testing result is much more likely to be wrong than right. (That said, conventional tests for environmental allergies are 85 percent accurate, which is encouraging.) Dr. Dodds' NutriScan test, which uses the pet's saliva and can be easily ordered by the pet owner, is an accurate test for food sensitivities. This is an excellent test, but it obviously leaves the pet owner with restricted dietary choices. Additionally, food sensitivities change over time, so you need to repeat the test twice a year.

Effective Microorganisms™

Effective Microorganisms™ (EM™) are a whole different can of worms (or should I say a whole different mix of microbes?). What is EM? Well, once upon a time, there was a man who wanted to heal the planet. He discovered an amazing combination of microorganisms that eliminated the need for pesticides and herbicides, cleared up lakes and rivers, cleaned up oil spills, and restored people and pets to good health. EM is a unique combination of beneficial microorganisms that operate in a revolutionary relationship with each other and, in so doing, make living organisms like plants, animals, and humans amazingly healthier.

The product was discovered by a Japanese horticulturalist, Dr. Teruo Higa, in the early 1980s. This dedicated doctor spent years researching microorganisms, trying to find the perfect combination of beneficial bacteria that would enhance the growth of plants without the need for toxic pesticides. He wanted to be able to make up for the damage that humans have inflicted on the earth with his soon-to-be-sought-after discovery.

After many years of examining thousands and thousands of microorganisms and discarding the bad ones, he was left with a cocktail of eighty strains of beneficial bacteria. Ironically, not knowing exactly what he had, he unceremoniously threw the mix on the back lawn outside his office and went away for a long weekend. Upon returning, he noticed that the patch of lawn onto which he threw the mixture was different than the surrounding area. It was greener and more vibrant, and, after just a few short days, looked much better than the rest of the lawn.

So what did this miracle mix actually contain? The solution contained *yeast, lactic acid bacteria,* and *phototrophic bacteria.* Yeast works to ferment foods and, in the process, creates amino acids

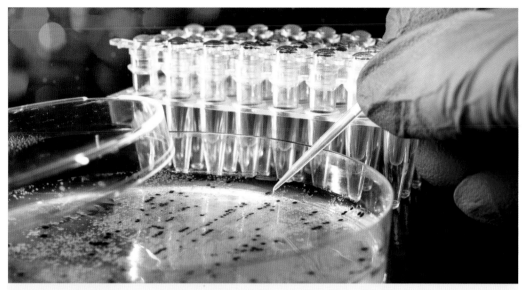
Ongoing research hopes to find new ways to help those affected by allergies.

Defense: Jaffe-Mellor Technique (JMT)

Holistic practitioners Carolyn Jaffe, D.Ac. Dipl. NCCA, and Judith Mellor, RN, identified mycoplasmas as the prime suspects in triggering a host of ailments, including many autoimmune diseases, and developed a revolutionary technique to reprogram an immune system that is destroying the body's tissues in its attempt to root out stealth invaders. The technique is called JMT, which stands for the Jaffe-Mellor Technique. JMT involves an advanced muscle-testing method, desensitization, deactivation, intervention, and acupressure.

Jaffe and Mellor's work has been invaluable to me in curing all kinds of autoimmune disease in my patients. Like Nambudripad's Allergy Elimination Techniques (NAET), JMT works to correct the reaction to the agent and rectify the confusion within the immune system. So when I treat to neutralize and eliminate allergies and food intolerances, I also utilize JMT to handle the mycoplasmas. The mycoplasmas are usually a very important culprit in the guts of animals with IBD, for which I choose a NAET-like allergy-elimination technique and JMT approach.

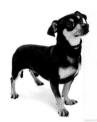
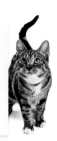

and polysaccharides, which become food for other microorganisms. It's commonly used to make bread. Lactic acid bacteria convert sugars into lactic acid and are used in cheese and yogurt. Ever since Louis Pasteur discovered lactic acid bacteria, they've been noted for their beneficial effects on health and longevity. Lactic acid bacteria also suppress harmful microorganisms and fungal growth. Lactic acid bacteria are also called (drum roll, please) *probiotics*.

The most extraordinary ingredients in this serendipitous gathering of microorganisms are the phototrophic bacteria. Phototrophic bacteria have actually been on this planet for a long, long time—since before there was oxygen. In fact, they're anaerobic, meaning that they live without oxygen. Phototrophic bacteria survive by using solar energy to metabolize organic and inorganic substances.

Most interestingly, before Earth had its present concentration of oxygen, these bacteria lived on carbon dioxide, ammonia, methane, and hydrogen sulfide, and they still do. What's *really* important is that these microbes thrive on poisons and pollutants—things that are excessively abundant on our planet today.

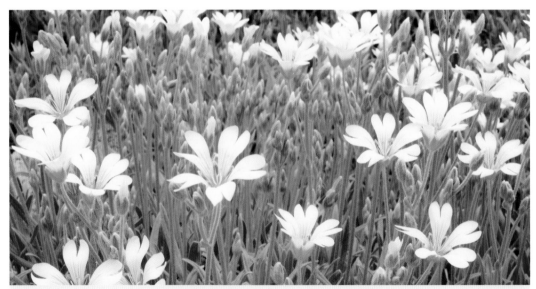

EM began as a way to eliminate pesticides from our gardens and crops.

The phototrophic bacteria, as we now know, consume carbon dioxide and other toxins and pollutants. Then, in a magical dance, these same microbes excrete oxygen, amino acids, antioxidants, and other substances that enhance life. It's truly a case of "in with the bad and out with the good."

No one had ever put these microbes together in this way before. The carbon dioxide produced by every oxygen-loving bacteria becomes food for the phototrophic bacteria, and the phototrophic bacteria then release oxygen for the rest of the bacteria. Everyone wins in this mix. But the real winners are your dogs and cats. The results have been nothing short of astounding.

EM is a product for humans that can also be used with pets. EM acts like a probiotic, but it's much more powerful. In both people and pets, most probiotic products are destroyed in the stomach before they ever make it to the intestinal tract, but EM survives to do its beneficial work.

I frequently treat pets with chronic diarrhea and irritable bowel disease with EM, and the results are dramatic. Think about a team of microorganisms that are thriving on the toxins and pollution in the digestive tract and generating antioxidants along with other super-healthy by-products while simultaneously overcoming the bad bugs in the gut.

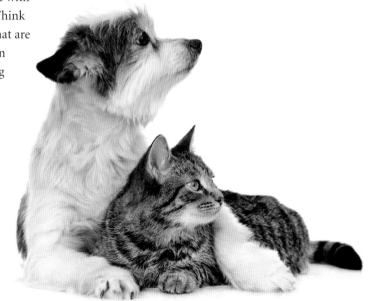

Thanks to Dr. Teruo Higa, who tried for years to find a magical mix of microbes that could help to heal our planet, we have a formulation that can help us all. The people, pets, and planet Dr. Higa loves so much all benefit spectacularly.

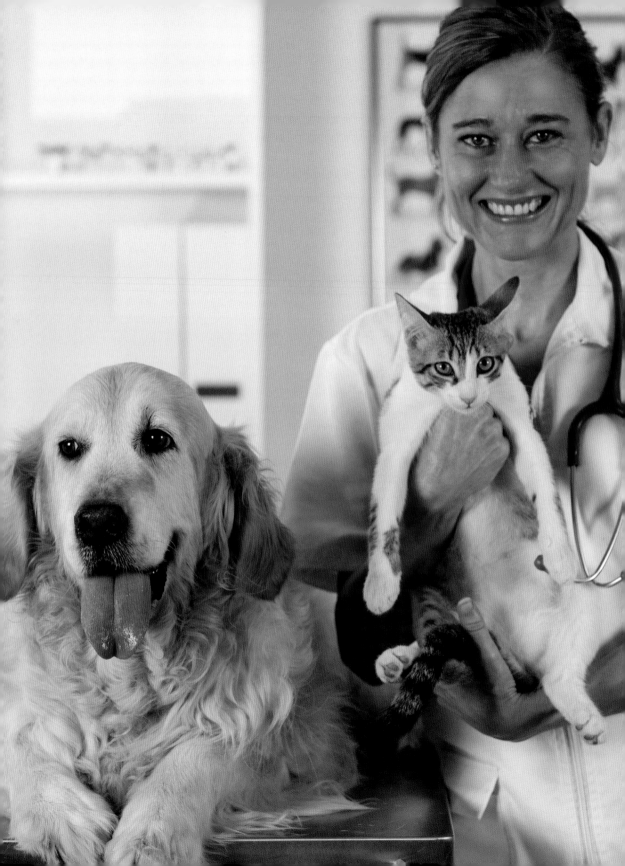

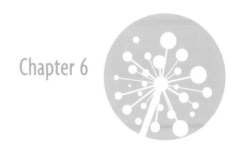

Chapter 6

Vetting Vaccines:
Separating Truth from Fiction

"A practice that was started many years ago and that lacks
scientific validity or verification is annual revaccination.
Almost without exception, there is no immunologic
requirement for annual revaccination. Immunity to viruses
persists for years in the life of the animal."

–Veterinary immunologist Ronald Schultz, PhD,
and Tom R. Phillips, DVM, PhD, in
Kirk's Current Veterinary Therapy XI

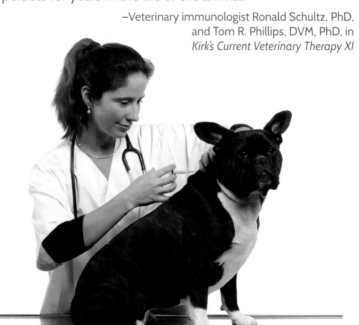

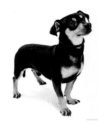

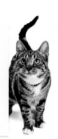

Did You Know?

Vaccines are highly implicated in contributing to the extraordinary increase in the amount of and severity of allergies in our dogs and cats.

This chapter about vaccinations is packed with information for you. And there's a very good reason for this: you need the facts so that you'll know the truth and have real knowledge about vaccinations and the inherent risks of overvaccination. The material in this chapter will arm you with dependable data and incontestable information, enabling you to make wise choices, discuss vaccines intelligently with your veterinarian, protect your pet's health, and even save money over the years.

So you've received your postcard from the vet's office, reminding you that it's vaccination time again. But didn't you just go through this same routine last year?

If your pet needs to be vaccinated so often, why, you might wonder, don't you need to have that polio vaccination you received as a baby repeated annually? How is it that animal control officers and veterinary students receive one rabies vaccine, and their blood tests show high immunity for

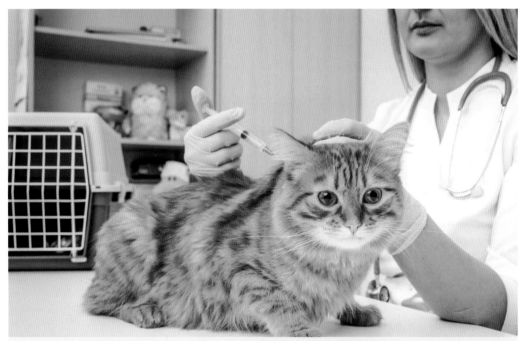

Many pet owners stick to regular vaccination schedules, but which shots are actually necessary?

the rest of their lives? While repeated rabies vaccines are necessary for compliance with the state you live in, many of your pet's vaccinations do not need to be given over and over and over again.

In the 1980s, allergies were relatively uncommon in pets. Now, the incidence of allergies in both dogs and cats has escalated into epidemic proportions. While a number of changes in the average pet's everyday life has occurred over the course of recent decades, one indisputable fact is overvaccination.

I guess one way to look at vaccines is that we're getting a lot more than we pay for. That's because vaccines contain all kinds of viruses in addition to the ones you think you're getting, along with extras like mycoplasmas and nanobacteria. Remember, vaccines also contain bits of chicken and cow from the chicken embryos and bovine serum that incubate them. Then, after injection, these food products are interpreted by the immune system as additional alien invaders. It's no coincidence, then, that the first foods usually eliminated from an allergic pet's diet are chicken and beef.

The rub is that most of the vaccinations you get the yearly reminder card for are not even necessary. That's why we have to learn which vaccines are really necessary and which ones are, pardon the expression, overkill. You want to give only the vaccines that are necessary and only as often as necessary.

Becoming an Expert on Vaccinations

If expert advice is what you need, be aware that many experts at prestigious veterinary schools are speaking out against the regimen of yearly vaccines as well as questioning the validity of giving certain vaccines at all. Before I share my own opinions, let's consider some of the official positions taken by various veterinary institutions.

- *Kirk's Current Veterinary Therapy IX*, a major reference book for veterinarians, states that the practice of giving annual vaccinations "lacks scientific validity or verification" and goes on to note that "immunity to viruses persists for years or for the life of the animal."
- In 2007, an American Veterinary Medical Association (AVMA) committee report stated that the annual revaccination recommendation frequently found on many vaccination labels is based on historical precedent, not scientific data.

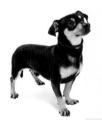
Did You Know?
Vaccines confuse our pets' immune systems and cause them to react inappropriately.
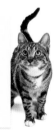

- Serology testing and challenge studies indicate that the duration of immunity for the canine distemper and canine parvovirus vaccines has been demonstrated to be a minimum of five to fifteen years. In fact, AVMA guidelines now accept that one additional puppy vaccine after eighteen weeks of age can protect a dog for life.

I recommend trying to hold off on puppy and kitten vaccinations until ten weeks of age. Puppies can get a distemper and parvovirus combination vaccine at ten, fourteen, and eighteen weeks, followed by a titer test at twenty-four weeks. If a puppy has a positive titer, he is protected for life. As far as kittens go, the same schedule of ten, fourteen, and eighteen weeks for the combination FVRCP vaccination provides lifetime protection; titer tests are not usually taken. If you have an indoor cat, she can be vaccinated at fourteen and eighteen weeks only. Or, if your cat is going to be indoors and isolated from any other cats, do you want to vaccinate her at all?

Much research demonstrates that my preferred approach is a valid approach to vaccination. It's been known for many decades that maternal antibodies can interfere with vaccinations given before ten weeks of age. Additionally, vaccines should be given three to four weeks apart—not two weeks apart—because the previous vaccine will interfere with the effectiveness of the subsequent vaccine if there is not enough time between vaccinations.

As a result of all of this research, most veterinary schools in North America have changed their protocols for vaccinating dogs and cats. These veterinary schools, along with the AVMA, have looked at studies that show how long vaccines last and have concluded that annual revaccination is unnecessary. Quite simply, there is no scientific documentation to support the supposed need for yearly vaccinations. At the same time, research shows that these same vaccinations subject your pets to the potential risks of allergic reactions and immune-mediated disease. Immunology expert Ronald Schultz, PhD, Diplomate ACVIM (American College of Veterinary Internal Medicine) has spent much of his career studying animal vaccines. Dr. Schultz is professor emeritus and former chair of the Department of Pathobiological Sciences at the University of Wisconsin-Madison School of Veterinary Medicine, and he has more than forty years of experience in the field of immunology.

According to Dr. Schultz, "The recommendation for annual revaccination is a practice that was officially started in 1978. This recommendation was made without any

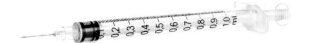

scientific validation of the need to booster immunity so frequently. The patient receives no benefit and may be placed at serious risk when an unnecessary vaccine is given."

The FVRCP vaccination contains feline viral rhinotracheitis, calicivirus, and panleukopenia (feline distemper). This is sometimes called the "yearly booster," even though it is not needed yearly. Kittens typically receive this vaccination after eight or ten weeks of age. As with dogs, studies show that a vaccination at or after eighteen weeks of age will protect a cat against feline distemper for life in just about every case. However, like the common cold in humans, there is no 100-percent effective vaccine in cats for calicivirus and herpes because viruses mutate, and there are many different strains.

There's also a link between the FVRCP vaccination and kidney inflammation because the vaccine contains feline kidney tissue, and this causes a low-level chronic inflammatory response. If you're curious about why so many cats over the age of ten have kidney problems, which eventually leads to kidney failure and death, you may be looking at the reason right now: the viruses used to make vaccines need to be grown in what is called a "cell culture," and the cells used to make the FVRCP vaccine are feline kidney cells.

When these kidney cells are injected (along with the vaccine) into the cat, her immune systems views them as foreign and makes antibodies against them. Unfortunately, those antibodies do not know the difference between the injected kidney cells and the cat's own kidney tissue, resulting in a potential autoimmune attack on the cat's kidneys (*auto* means "self"). So that's another argument in favor of minimal vaccinations.

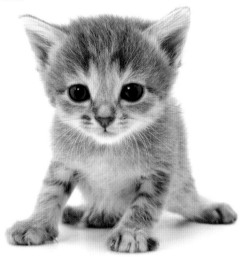

The rabies vaccination in cats, as in dogs, is also a legal requirement. Rabies is a very serious disease with a high mortality rate. Bat rabies is the most common strain to infect humans and pets. For our cats, considering the risk of vaccine-induced sarcoma (malignant tumor at the injection site), I recommend a nonadjuvanted (live) vaccine, such as Merial's PureVax™ rabies vaccination. Not all vets carry the three-year vaccine, but you will want the three-year, rather than the annual, vaccine for your cat. I also recommend the IMRAB® 3 TF rabies vaccination by Merial. It is a thimerosal-free formulation that provides three years of rabies protection to dogs and cats.

I hope you're getting my point that you can stop vaccinating your pet every year. The kitten or puppy vaccines work just fine to protect your pet for life if given after eighteen weeks of age. A blood test called a *titer test* can prove that your pet has immunity. If you're the nervous type, you can give one more FVRCP booster to your cat or one distemper/parvo booster to your dog at one year and five months of age, and that's all your pet would need for those particular vaccines.

Perhaps after reading about the medical problems that vaccines can promote and cause, you'll stick with titer tests and stand your ground on vaccinations when interacting with your veterinarian. You won't be exposing your pets to the possible complications of overvaccination.

Weapons of Overvaccination

Before vaccines became an annual ritual (around the 1970s), the incidence of allergies, autoimmune disease, and cancer in the canine population was a mere fraction of what it is today. Since then, vaccine producers have encouraged the veterinary establishment to use their products whenever possible, and, as a result, the manufacture of pet vaccinations has evolved into multibillion-dollar enterprise.

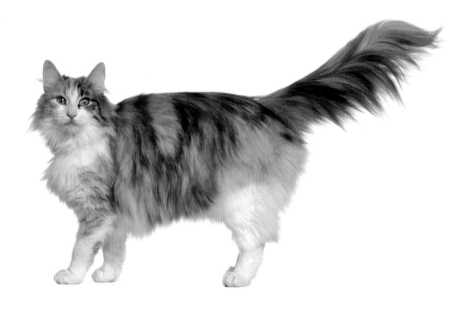

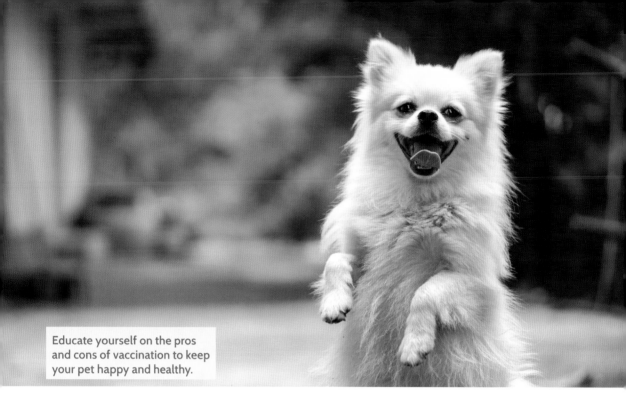

Educate yourself on the pros and cons of vaccination to keep your pet happy and healthy.

Vaccine manufacturers have also been successful at something else: evading responsibility for the damage that their products can cause. Vaccine companies have become indemnified. This means that you can't sue the manufacturer if your pet becomes severely ill or dies due to a vaccination or related complications, although occasionally a company may reimburse a pet owner's medical expenses to demonstrate the "good will" of the company.

Our pets' immune systems, created millions of years ago, were never designed to cope with the multiple diseases that are injected, all at once, into their bodies. Vaccinations can cause many long-term medical problems, including behavior problems. The more often you give these vaccines, the greater the opportunity for these illnesses to establish themselves in your pet.

I've treated allergies in dogs and cats for around forty years. People have come from other states, often traveling a long way, to have me evaluate, diagnose, and treat their pets' allergies, but they would see their local veterinarians for physical exams and routine issues. I've very often seen cured pets regress into their previous allergic state after receiving (unnecessary) annual boosters from their local vets. I would then have to go through the allergy fix again with the pets and their owners, which incurs costs and time, all because of vaccines that were probably not necessary at all.

Again and again, I've seen what vaccines can do to both dogs and cats. In fact, there are entire books written on the subject. Suffice it to say, if these vaccines were needed to protect our pets against the ravages of severe diseases, they might be warranted. But when the dog or cat is protected by a vaccine administered when he or she was a young pup or kitten, the situation becomes a travesty. Vaccines play an important role in the development of allergies in our pets, and there are also are many other reasons why we want to be sparing in the use of vaccinations with our fine furry friends.

Vaccine Contamination and a New Disease

When I entered veterinary school in 1976, parvovirus in dogs didn't exist. No dogs were presented to the University of Pennsylvania School of Veterinary Medicine with parvovirus until 1978. During my senior year, I observed case after case of canines with life-threatening, bloody diarrhea. They were admitted to ICU and placed on supportive IV fluids under twenty-four-hour care.

Canine parvovirus type 2 (CPV2) appeared simultaneously around the world and killed millions of dogs in Australia, Europe, Asia, and the United States. At the time of the outbreak, this brand-new disease didn't seem to be spreading from one dog to another. World health professionals wondered how the disease could be traveling around the world so quickly. They found their answer.

You see, this new disease was being delivered to each dog in his yearly booster shot. Batches of vaccines had been shipped to veterinarians all over the world. And, no, the vaccine companies were not anticipating this disease and adding CPV2 just for good measure. In those days, the booster shots would have included distemper, hepatitis, leptospirosis, and parainfluenza; there was no such thing as a DHLPP.

Here's the inside scoop. The canine vaccine stocks had long been contaminated with a feline virus. Remember, a vaccine contains the viruses from which it protects your dog, but it also contains components that you didn't ask for and don't want. The sudden and devastating outbreak of CPV2 happened because the feline panleukopenia virus (FPV), which had long been present in

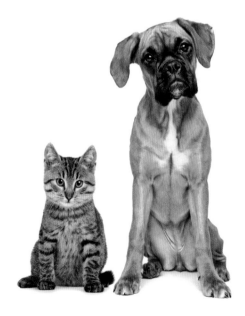

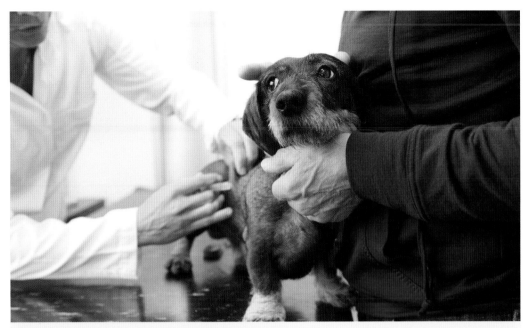
Parvovirus is now one of the core vaccines for dogs.

dog vaccines, mutated into a form that could jump species and infect dogs! It makes sense that the symptoms of feline panleukopenia are very similar to parvovirus symptoms in dogs.

So, what did the vaccine companies do? They figured that they had to immunize dogs fast, so they began to sell the actual FPV vaccine as a CPV2 vaccination for dogs. The virus in the cat vaccine, unlike the unwelcome contaminant virus in the dog vaccine, had not yet learned to jump species.

Dogs were being vaccinated en masse with the FPV vaccine about eight weeks before my second clinical round in ICU. This time, it was different. Instead of parvovirus patients, the ICU was filled with dogs with autoimmune hemolytic anemia. And they all contracted their autoimmune disease about six to eight weeks after their feline vaccination. Coincidence?

Vaccine-Associated Sarcomas (VAS)

My alma mater was the first to recognize VAS in cats in 1991. Highly aggressive and deadly fibrosarcoma tumors were between cats' shoulder blades, exactly where the rabies vaccines were commonly injected. In those days, veterinary students were taught to change the injection site for cat's rabies vaccination to a hind leg because a leg could be easily amputated if a VAS formed.

VAS is commonly seen in cats. Dogs can also get VAS at vaccination sites, but it's not nearly as common. Nowadays, in the case of tail-wagging dogs, many veterinary schools are advocating that vets give the rabies vaccination at the end of the tail—again, because it is easy to amputate.

Problem solved? Not really. First of all, I don't know of any veterinarians who give rabies vaccinations in the tail. Second, all this does is simply amplify how critical the situation has become.

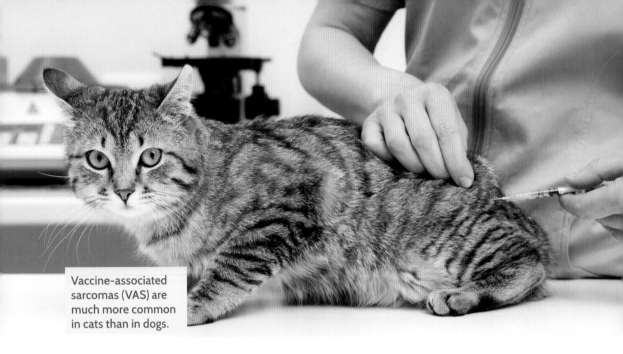

Vaccine-associated sarcomas (VAS) are much more common in cats than in dogs.

Fibrosarcoma is the most common VAS cancer from a rabies vaccination. Other tumor types include rhabdomyosarcoma, myxosarcoma, chondrosarcoma, malignant histiocytoma, and undifferentiated sarcoma.

All of these types of cancer are characterized as highly invasive, rapidly growing, and malignant. Often, the cancer spreads to the lungs and may spread to the regional lymph nodes as well.

So it's not just allergies. Vaccines can also be the direct causes of many fatal diseases in addition to chronic diseases.

Rabies vaccines are legal requirements in many states, but the AVMA has passed guidelines allowing veterinarians to temporarily exempt pets from rabies vaccinations in certain circumstances, including for medical reasons. Chronic allergies or chronic diarrhea can certainly be categorized as an illness. If your veterinarian writes a letter to exempt your pet from vaccination due to illness, and your town's health department accepts it, you can hold off on the vaccination. If you want to be extra careful, you can take a titer test to reassure yourself that your pet has retained immunity.

What Vaccines Does Your Pet Really Need?

Each vaccine is different in its protection and efficacy. For instance, the kennel cough vaccine does not actually protect against the disease; it simply works to lessen the severity of the disease. Because you're vaccinating for a bacteria in this case, you would actually need to vaccinate four times each year because the duration of limited immunity is only three months. When you consider the fact that kennel cough is a self-limiting upper respiratory problem that responds rapidly to homeopathic remedies and colloidal silver, it seems a bit ridiculous to give your dog this "yearly" vaccination (which only really lasts for three months). That said, many groomers, doggy

Do Not Mix!

Please do not mix vaccines. They all contain adjuvants and substances other than the viral or bacterial components, and that adds up to a greater likelihood of adverse reactions. Dogs should get the rabies vaccine at a separate time from the distemper and parvo vaccines; distemper and parvo come as a combined injection, and they are fine to get at the same time. Our feline friends should get the FVRCP vaccine at a separate time from the rabies vaccination.

daycares, and boarding kennels require it. If you use a mobile groomer rather than going to a grooming salon, and an in-home dog sitter rather than a boarding kennel, you can avoid giving this vaccination.

The distemper/parvo and FVCRP vaccinations are considered the *core vaccines*. There are many other vaccinations such as Lyme disease, leptospirosis, canine influenza, feline infectious peritonitis (FIP), feline immunodeficiency virus (FIV), and feline leukemia (FeLV) vaccinations that are *not* core vaccinations and should *not* be administered routinely. In the appendix of this book, you will find more detailed explanations of core vaccinations for dogs and cats, the benefits and risks of noncore vaccinations for both species, and information on the AVMA vaccination guidelines.

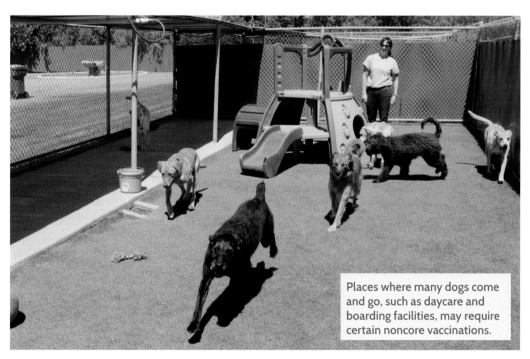

Places where many dogs come and go, such as daycare and boarding facilities, may require certain noncore vaccinations.

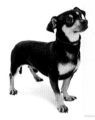

Did You Know?

When measuring a dog's or cat's protection against disease, renowned pet-vaccination expert Dr. Ronald Schultz believes that once a test yields strong titers, you need not test again.

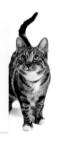

By this point, I sincerely hope that you have become knowledgeable about vaccines and that you understand the dangers of overvaccination, which is rampant in veterinary medicine today. The only way to handle this aspect of your pet's care is to become more informed and, as far as vaccinations go, to take your pet's health into your own hands.

Titer Testing

I've mentioned titer tests several times already, but a more detailed discussion here is warranted. A titer test is a laboratory test that measures the presence and level of antibodies to disease in the blood. Antibodies are produced when an antigen (such as a canine or feline distemper virus) provokes a response from the immune system. This response can come from natural exposure or from vaccination.

Titer testing requires testing a small amount of your pet's blood. Some veterinarians now offer in-office titer tests that can be done while you and your pet are at the clinic for an examination. Other titer tests are done by outside laboratories, in which case your veterinarian will draw and send out your pet's blood. Alternatively, you can send the blood in yourself and work directly with Jean Dodds, DVM, at Hemopet (*www.hemopet.org*), but your veterinarian will still need to draw the blood for you. Additionally, Dr. Ronald Schultz tests titers at the School of Veterinary Medicine at the University of Wisconsin-Madison.

Quite honestly, if your dog has been vaccinated for parvovirus or distemper or if your cat has been vaccinated for distemper (panleukopenia) after his or her first year of life, your pet will be more than likely to hold that immunity for life. However, you may want the peace of mind of testing your pet every three to five years. Interestingly, more dog owners than cat owners have titer tests done, and that's not because their cats are second-class citizens! It's just that cat owners are more comfortable with their cats' retained immunity if they had vaccinations after eighteen weeks of age—just like you don't bother getting a titer test for that polio shot you had when you were two years old.

The most useful time to run a titer test is after your youngster has received his or her initial series of vaccinations, especially if you've limited that series to just one or two vaccinations, the last being after sixteen weeks of age. It's likely that you've conferred lifetime immunity to your pet with these two vaccinations alone. Dogs and cats who have had one or more yearly boosters after their first birthdays should be set for life, and a titer test is likely a waste of your money.

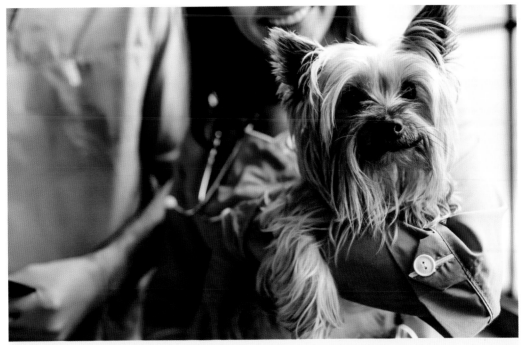

Titer tests can reveal if your pet will have sufficient protection without additional boosters.

If a titer test reveals any measurable titer to the disease(s) in question, you've achieved your goal: your pet has actively made immunity to the viruses with which he or she was vaccinated. The test results don't need to meet some minimum standard of protection; they just have to be positive. Positive titer results indicate that you are likely now the proud owner of an immune pet, and you can confidently decline further vaccines. For how long? For life.

Remember: If you give a second or third parvo/distemper vaccination after eighteen weeks of age to your puppy, the immunity will likely last for life; the same holds true for kittens and the FVCRP vaccine. Add a booster a year later, at one year and eighteen weeks of age, and you can feel secure that your dog or cat is protected for life. Still concerned? Have one titer test done to confirm lifetime protection. (See Appendix II for more details.)

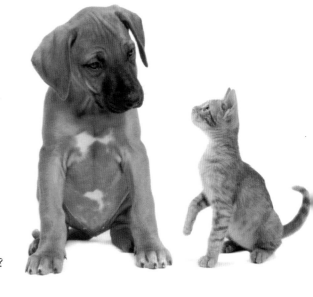

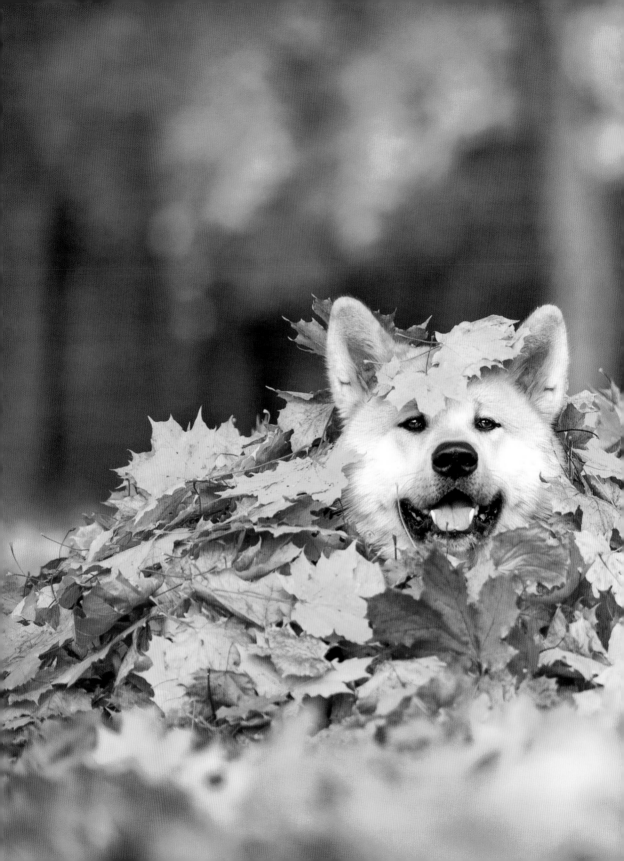

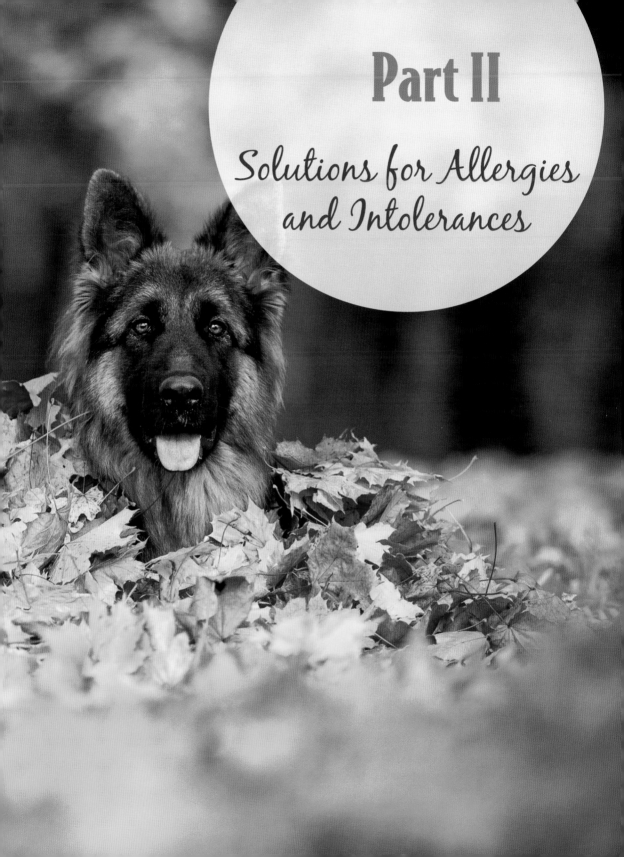

Part II

Solutions for Allergies and Intolerances

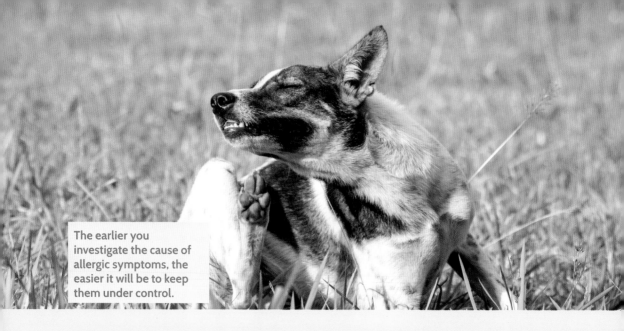

The earlier you investigate the cause of allergic symptoms, the easier it will be to keep them under control.

The Need for a New Approach

Root causes aside, the thing to remember about allergies and food sensitivities is that they tend to intensify and widen with time unless you take aggressive measures to nip them in the bud. A pet who develops an itch for a couple of weeks in the summertime might be tormented for the entire summer the following year, with the condition growing progressively worse until it is a year-round problem. The same goes for gastrointestinal problems, which are prevalent in both dogs and cats.

Because allergies and food sensitivities/intolerances are becoming all too common, we have to think about preventing these problems whether we get a puppy or kitten or adopt an older pet. We already know that frequent exposure, year after year, to vaccines that your pet never needed in the first place has a vital role in exacerbating and worsening allergies, so the simple advice here is to avoid overvaccination.

We know that allergies, insensitivities, and intolerances are due to an overactive, confused immune system. We also know that vaccinations create a situation in which the immune system is overwhelmed. When a virus attacks a body in a normal manner, the immune response is elegantly orchestrated. With vaccines, the shock of the unnatural influx of multiple viruses knocks the whole immune system out of whack, and this inflammatory response doesn't fade away—it persists, and it has a hair trigger.

Remember, the best way for an allergy or sensitivity to develop and worsen is through repeated and frequent exposure to something, and this holds true for both vaccinations and diet. By varying your pet's diet, you'll not only provide him with more balanced nutrition, but you'll also reduce the opportunity for food allergies to develop. Conventional kibble can perpetuate the allergy cycle when consumed regularly if it contains dyes, preservatives, and poor-quality proteins that can serve as red flags to a malfunctioning immune system. A varied diet will also allow you to isolate and remove those items to which your pet might be allergic.

A Swedish study showed that children who were supplemented with a vitamin/mineral mix had significantly fewer incidences of allergies than children who did not receive a supplement. I readily assume that this is also true for dogs and cats, so start supplementing your puppies and kittens early on with a complete and balanced product. I recommend Deserving Pets' Canine Everyday Essentials for dogs and Vital Vities for cats. Both are microencapsulated to protect the ingredients from oxidation and degradation.

Keep in mind that the intensity of an allergy might be the result of a synergistic effect of two or more allergens combining. Your pet might have a severe allergic reaction to yeast, for instance, and mild reactions to corn, wheat, and soy. And while you might make a point of not feeding him anything that contains yeast, a food that contains the other three ingredients might produce a reaction that is just as, if not more, severe. The fact that these three ingredients are present together will increase the allergic response even though the individual allergy to each of them is not nearly as severe as the one triggered by yeast. The bottom line is that the number of allergens in your pet's environment plus the intensity of the allergy to each equals the total allergic reaction.

It's incredibly important to minimize the amount of toxins and poisons our dogs and cats encounter in everyday life. After my many years of practice, it is my firm opinion that toxic exposure is *surely* causing allergies, cancer, and many other illnesses. So, with the aim of keeping our pets healthier, let's dive into some information about the toxins to which our pets exposed, followed by discussions on allergy "copycats," and then preventive measures and solutions for allergies and intolerances.

Regarding solutions, we're going to work to correct your pet's immune dysfunction and set him or her back on a path to health. You'll have many different options available to you, including homeopathic remedies, Chinese herbs, and other natural products along with diet change. My favorite is the Allergy Elimination 4 Pets technique, a method that I have used for decades in treating chronic GI problems, such as IBD, and itchy skin problems caused by food sensitivities and general allergies.

Did You Know?

As Benjamin Franklin said, "An ounce of prevention is worth a pound of cure," and it's never too early to start working to prevent allergies in your dogs and cats by reducing or eliminating the common causes: vaccines, toxins, chemicals, and poor diet.

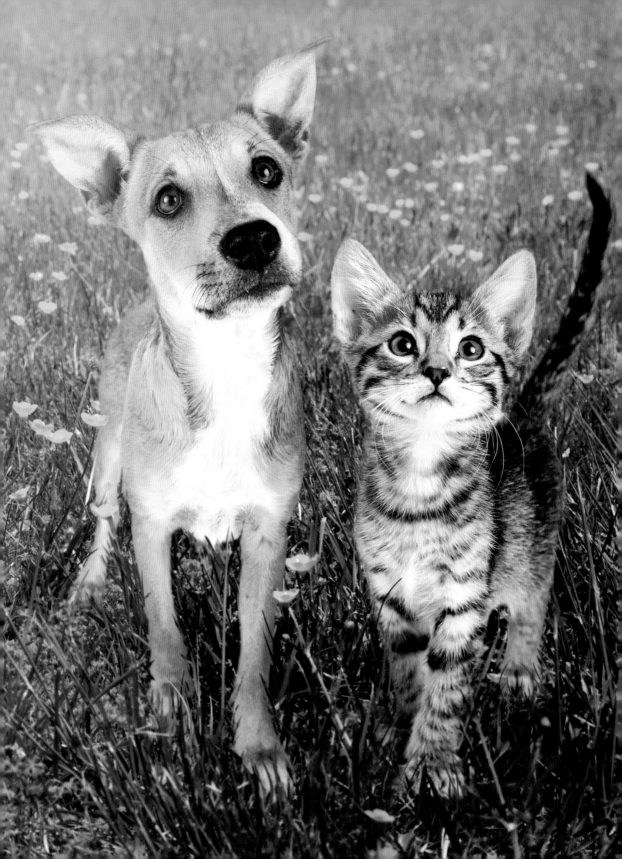

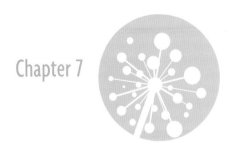

Chapter 7

Flea and Tick Prevention: Protection Does Not Have to Poison

> "Under our free institutions, anybody can poison himself that wants to and will pay the price."
>
> –Mark Twain

I remember when my twins were eight years old, and there was a lice problem at their school. Parents would rather shave their kids' heads than shampoo just *once* with the toxic product that's commonly used to eliminate lice. And these parents weren't even holistically motivated! Why aren't we thinking this way with our pets? Folks give their pets spot-on and oral preventives for fleas and ticks, basically making them poison-soaked sponges of insecticide. Flea and tick products are toxic— and this is *proven by research*.

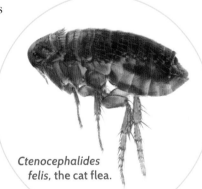

Ctenocephalides felis, the cat flea.

Some products boast that they start killing fleas and ticks twenty minutes after they're applied. Some are effective for ninety days. We all seem to trust the drug companies, so we don't wonder how a product that stays inside our pets day after day, week after week, and even month after month could possibly be healthy for them.

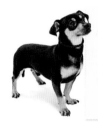

Did You Know?

Vaccines are highly implicated in contributing to the extraordinary increase in the amount of and severity of allergies in our dogs and cats.

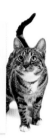

In my years as a holistic veterinarian, I've come across a fair share of people who are head over heels in love with their pets. I, too, am guilty as charged. Nonetheless, I've discovered a troublesome propensity for folks to faithfully administer spot-on flea and tick preventives no matter the time of year or the likelihood of the pet to pick up either of these parasites.

Because we love our pets, we want what's best for them. None of us wants our pets to get one of those nasty tick-borne diseases. But unquestioningly administering harsh chemicals for flea and tick prevention is not what's actually best for them. These chemicals go right through and into your pet's internal systems, indisputably increasing his or her risk of cancer, allergies, and many other diseases. The poison in these products circulates throughout your pet at levels high enough to kill a flea or tick just as soon as the pest bites and reaches blood. Your pet essentially retains the residue of insecticide and becomes a poison bomb after you spot-treat him.

Evaluate the Situation

Flea and tick prevention is not a "one-size-fits-all" formula. Every family pet has a particular lifestyle. Let's say it's summertime, and you have three small dogs who play and romp in your securely fenced yard, rarely meeting other dogs. The chances of these dogs getting fleas and ticks

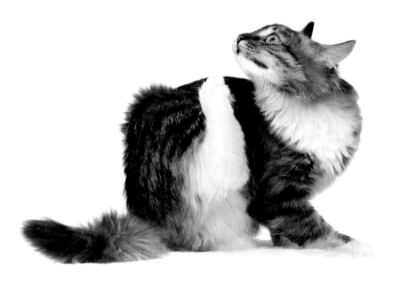

A Look at Heartworm Preventives

Heartworm disease is transmitted by mosquitoes. Only the female is capable of transmission. She lives for fourteen days, and, during this time, she has to find and bite an infected dog to become infective herself. Heartworm medication works backward, killing the young larvae that may have infected your dog up to forty-five days earlier. So the word "preventive" is a bit of a misnomer—although it does prevent adult heartworms from infecting the dog, the drugs actually kill the larvae.

You may want to assess your dog's heartworm risk and dose accordingly. Visit the American Heartworm Society's website (*www.heartwormsociety.org*) and take a look at the heartworm incidence maps for the United States to see how prevalent heartworm really is in your area of the country. Use this information to decide if you want to treat your dog with heartworm preventive. For example, those of us who live in northern areas certainly do not have to give the preventive in the dead of winter, when there are no mosquitoes.

are low. You can simply routinely check them and avoid using any toxic preventives. If the same three dogs plus two cats live in a household in Florida, fleas are a year-round problem for them, while ticks are not very common. Now, let's put those same three dogs and two cats in upstate New York and add long grass and proximity to deer. In this situation, ticks will be a problem.

What about in winter? Many dog owners continue to give flea and tick prevention (along with heartworm prevention) during snowy winters just for good measure. These dogs continue to be soaked in serious chemicals when nary a mosquito, tick, or flea is around in cold winter weather.

Are Spot-Ons Safe?

We don't want our pets to get fleas and ticks, and, more importantly, we want to avoid tick-borne diseases. So we give our dogs and cats chemical preventives that stay in their systems for months. The concentration of these insecticides in the animal's body is so high that even at the end of the one-month (or three-month, depending on the preventive) period, a flea or tick drops dead within seconds of nibbling on your pet. Even more interesting, though, are the poisons circulating through your pet's body day in and day out and how carcinogenic they are; the danger of these ingredients has been established repeatedly through research.

"Better safe than sorry" does not work in regard to the routine application of these very toxic products to our pets. It's time for us to learn just how dangerous spot-on products really are. In 2009 the Environmental Protection Agency (EPA) began reviewing the safety of spot-on flea and tick products, and what they found was not at all pretty.

One company's website states that the topical insecticide fipronil is absorbed into the sebaceous glands of the pet's skin, creating the impression that fipronil does not migrate into your pet's body, which is simply not true. Virginia Dobozy, VMD, MPH, of the EPA's Pesticide Division did a study tracing radioactive fipronil, and she found it in the fat, organs, urine, and feces of all exposed dogs. Tests show that, even at low doses, fipronil has the potential for nervous-system, liver, and thyroid toxicity; altered thyroid hormone levels; thyroid and other cancers; kidney damage; convulsions, loss of hair at or beyond the point of application; moist inflammation; and chemical burns and itching.

Another commonly used spot-on ingredient, imidacloprid, is a systemic insecticide belonging to a class of chemicals called the neonicotinoids. In laboratory studies, imidacloprid was found to cause thyroid lesions, liver toxicity, and increased cholesterol levels, and it has the potential for damaging the kidneys, liver, thyroid, heart, lungs, spleen, adrenal glands, brain, and gonads. As a neurotoxin, it caused weakened coordination, labored breathing, and muscle weakness. After its introductions in 1994, this drug was found to cause an increase in frequency of birth defects when tested on mice, rats, and dogs.

Most folks consider the natural alternative—pyrethrins (naturally occurring compounds from the chrysanthemum plant) and pyrethroids and permethrins (the synthetic counterparts)—as less hazardous. In fact, the contrary has been irrefutably

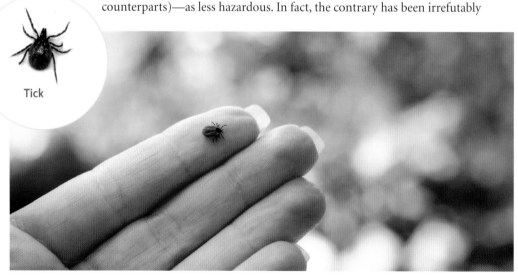

Tick

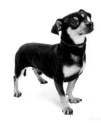

Did You Know?

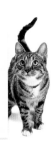

A chemical pharmaceutical product that kills fleas and ticks without adversely affecting your pet's health does not exist.

proven. Information released through the Freedom of Information Act to the Washington-based Center for Public Integrity (CPI) showed that from 2002 through 2007, at least 1,600 pet deaths from pyrethroid spot-on treatments were reported to the EPA. That's nearly double the number of reported fatalities linked to the other compounds. Pyrethroid spot-ons also accounted for more than half of "major" pesticide pet reactions, including brain damage, heart attacks, and seizures. And how many deaths and complications went unreported?

New pharmaceutical products to prevent fleas and ticks, whether oral, spot-on, or in collar form, contain higher concentrations of the same ingredients or even more dangerous compounds with far more serious side effects.

Some flea and tick products also add ingredients that prevent heartworms and kill intestinal worms. Think about the multiple doses of poisonous insecticides and chemicals that such products deliver all at one time, and on a routine basis. I have never met a dog or cat who needs an intestinal

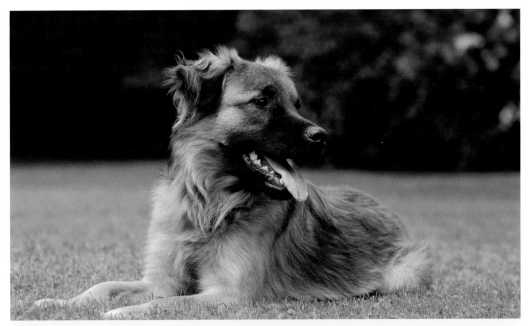

Both parasites and traditional parasite preventatives carry some risks for your pet.

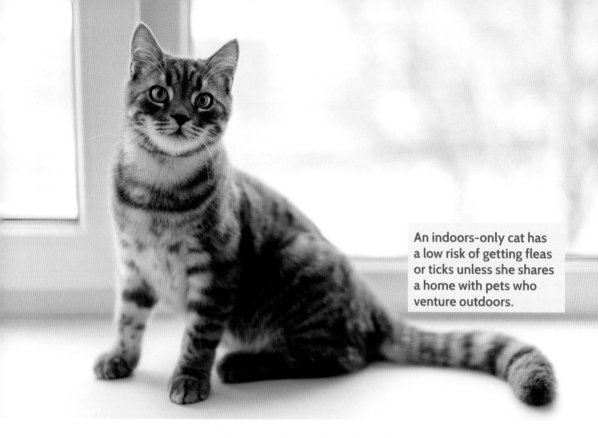

An indoors-only cat has a low risk of getting fleas or ticks unless she shares a home with pets who venture outdoors.

worming every month! Advertisements tell you about chewable preventives that start working within hours of ingestion and protect your pet from fleas and ticks for a month—or even three months! Manufacturers say that these products work from the inside out, and they certainly do—by soaking into all of your pet's internal systems.

The Risks

First of all, you need to assess how likely or unlikely your pet is to get ticks or fleas. One option is to do nothing and watch what happens. At the same time, be prepared to mobilize the minute you see a flea or tick. Fleas are by far the easiest pests to deal with naturally. Deserving Pets' Ticked Off! is a safe, all-natural product that dependably kills fleas, flea larvae, and flea eggs immediately. All you have to do is spray your pet along with the home environment and bedding, and the fleas are gone. It contains hydrolyzed silica, which works by suffocating the pests. Another product, called Herbal Defense Spray by Petzlife™, is an effective, natural solution for fleas and ticks. The manufacturer also makes an ingestible powder that you add to your pet's food high-tick areas.

If you live in a high-tick area, you need to make it a habit to routinely check your pets for ticks. If you find a tick, you must remove it ASAP. One method I really like is to pour rubbing alcohol into the bottle cap and invert the cap over the tick for thirty seconds, pressing the cap into the skin. You will find the dead tick floating in the liquid in the cap.

Notes on Garlic

· A large dog can have up to two small cloves of garlic per day, and a medium-sized dog can have up to one small clove of garlic a day.

· Garlic is not recommended for cats.

· The garlic essence comes out in the oil of a dog's fur to repel pests. If you're using garlic to help prevent fleas and ticks, always wash your dog with a detergent-free shampoo, such as castile soap shampoo, so you don't strip the garlic essence out of the fur.

Garlic, when fed to dogs (but not to cats), may help a bit in preventing both fleas and ticks. There are many products on the market containing garlic for this very purpose.

On the topic of garlic, it affords a multitude of health benefits, so don't believe the negative hype about garlic. Garlic is approved as a flavoring for use in dog food. Of garlic's reputed benefits, perhaps the best known is its use as a natural antibiotic, with evidence going back through history. Garlic has a broad-spectrum antibacterial effect, and, importantly, bacteria don't seem to build up a resistance to garlic.

But that's not all. Garlic increases the immune activity of killer cells, which are types of white blood cells that destroy infected and cancerous cells. Not every dog bitten by an infected tick will get a tick-borne disease. The state of that dog's immune system will decide if the infection takes hold. The antibacterial and immune-boosting action of garlic can save the day for your dog.

Furthermore, reported adverse affects from garlic add up to a total nonevent over a span of twenty-two years. The National Animal Supplement Council (www.nasc.cc) responsibly records both Adverse Events and Serious Adverse Events resulting from the use of natural products. A Serious Adverse Event is defined as: "An Adverse Event with a transient incapacitating effect (i.e., rendering the animal unable to function normally for a short period of time, such as with a seizure) or non-transient (i.e., permanent) health effect." Nine hundred million doses of garlic over twenty-two years resulted in only two Serious Adverse Events, and these episodes could very well have been due not to garlic but to another ingredient in the mix. This proves beyond a shadow of a doubt that the risk of using garlic is so low that it's statistically insignificant.

You now have alternatives to toxic spot-on and oral flea and tick products that you know will work. It's no secret that minimizing the toxins to which our pets are exposed will reduce their risk of cancer along with many other diseases. Because there are now natural products that are reliable and effective, there's no reason to have to use toxic products on your dog or cat.

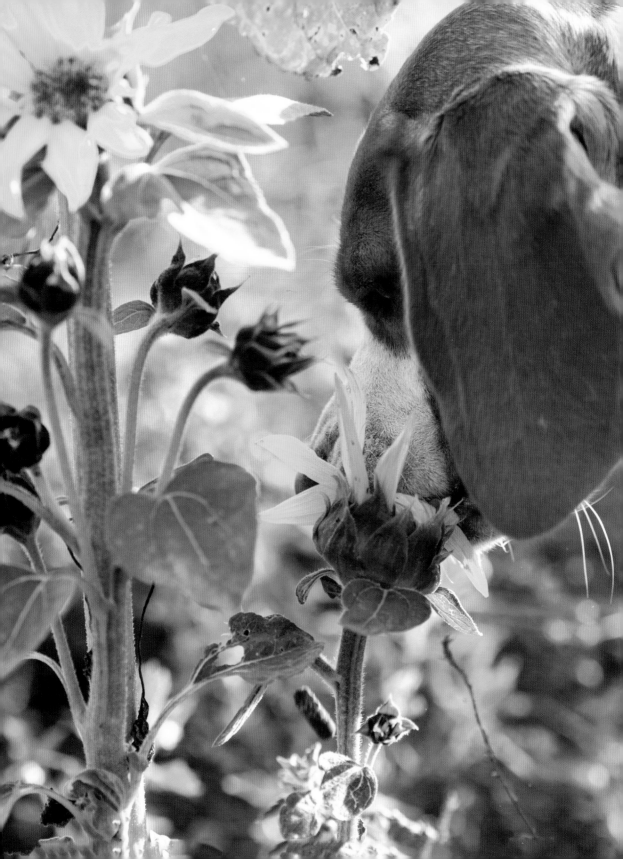

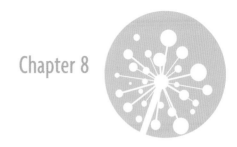

Chapter 8

Environmental Toxins: Fighting the Dangers around Our Pets

While we can control how often we vaccinate our pets as well as our use of chemical products, we can't really control all of the environmental toxins to which our pets are exposed. For hundreds of thousands of years, during the course of both human and canine evolution, changes occurred much more slowly in the natural environment than they do in our polluted world of today. The pesticides, herbicides, preservatives, colorings, and additives that we exposing our dogs and cats to are filling their bodies with residues that are totally alien to their systems.

One example is xenohormones, a group of either naturally occurring or artificially created compounds with hormone-like properties. They're frequently implicated in endocrine disruption, and it's the man-made types that can cause health problems in our pets.

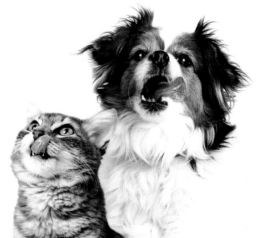

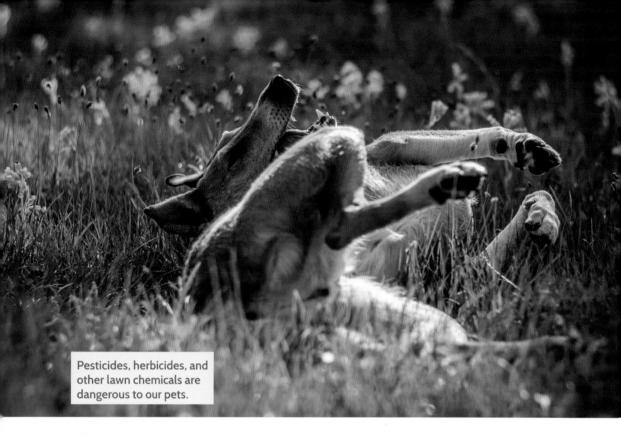

Pesticides, herbicides, and other lawn chemicals are dangerous to our pets.

Xenoestrogens are a type of xenohormone that imitates estrogen. These foreign exogenous hormones, unknown to man or beast until around the 1960s, mimic real hormones. In the body, they disrupt healthy processes and create disease. Our dogs and cats can be exposed to xenoestrogens from commercially raised, nonorganic meats, such as beef, chicken, and pork, along with commercial dairy products, including milk, butter, cheese, and ice cream.

To avoid xenoestrogens, you would have to use only organic products that do not contain bovine growth hormone. Nonfood products, such as dryer sheets and fabric softeners, also contain xenoestrogens along with other chemical toxins.

Herbicides containing glyphosate, a very potent xenoestrogen, are commonly sprayed all over the place, and they stay in the environment, leaving a residue where they were sprayed. When it rains, the herbicides become incorporated into a mist that rises a few feet from the ground. Our pets walk right through that mist. Exposure to glyphosate increases the risk of cancer. In fish, glyphosate herbicides have caused genetic damage and immune-system damage. In frogs, glyphosate herbicides caused genetic damage and abnormal development. In both fish and frogs, this chemical caused males to become females.

While we all know that limiting exposure to chemicals, pesticides, and toxins reduces the risk of cancer in our pets, we often forget about lawn care. Lawn chemicals have been shown to increase the risk of both bladder cancer and lymphosarcoma in dogs based on studies of these specific types of cancer. I would submit that lawn chemicals, in general, increase the risk of many types of cancer.

As with herbicides, lawn chemicals actually rise up into a fine mist that hangs a few feet over the lawn when it rains. Many of us think that the rain just washes these chemicals right into the soil, but this is definitely not the case. Our pets run through this toxic mist, inhaling the chemicals into their lungs and soaking them in through their feet. Every time they run around outside at home and in parks (which is more of a concern for dog owners than cat owners), more carcinogens enter their systems.

Certain cleaning products and particularly deodorizers are not healthy for your pets. Fabric softeners, dryer sheets, and room/carpet deodorizers should be totally avoided. White vinegar is a marvelous natural fabric softener with no smell after it dries. Simple baking soda is both safe and effective as a cleaning product; you can formulate healthy household cleaners with vinegar and baking soda. Remember, our pets are lying on those carpets and furniture, so you should seek safe alternatives to chemical-based sprays and powders, which are definitely not good for our pets' health.

Many labels on cleaning and other household products do not correctly represent all of the ingredients. In fact, a recent investigation of fourteen commonly used air fresheners by the Natural Resources Defense Council (NRDC) found hormone-disrupting chemicals known as phthalates in twelve of the products, including some that were marketed as "all-natural" and "unscented." None of the air fresheners listed phthalates on their labels. Further, many products are fragranced with coal tar oil; coal tar is a carcinogen that results from the burning of coal, and coal contains many compounds, including hydrocarbons and phenols.

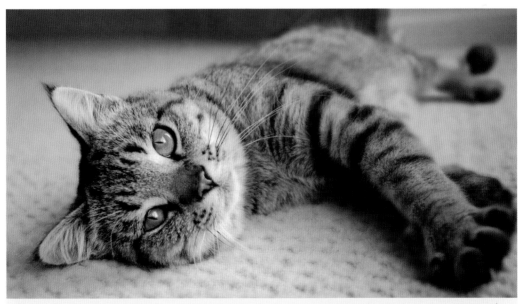

Chemicals used inside the home, such as carpet cleaners and deodorizers, also pose risks to pets.

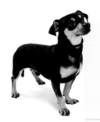

Did You Know?

Health is actually defined by the cell's ability to detoxify and repair itself.

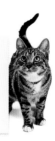

Detoxification and Diet

With every passing decade, the number and concentration of carcinogens to which our pets are exposed increases, and it's no wonder that the occurrence of cancer in pets has increased likewise. While it's impossible to avoid every carcinogen, we can certainly work to decrease the amount of toxins in our pets' environments and help strengthen their immune systems.

However, our pets can't live in bubbles. That's why it's important to give them daily supplements that help with detoxification. A good supplement should contain extra vitamin C along with the phytonutrients in vegetables such as kale, which dump toxins almost ten times faster from cells. Canine Everyday Essentials, by Deserving Pets (*www.deservingpets.com*), is a pure, highly bioactive, human-grade supplement that contains many detoxing vitamins, minerals, and phytonutrients from plants. Chlorophyll is also great to use as part of a daily detox routine.

Your pet's diet is the single most important factor for his or her health, immunity, and longevity. That's because particular foods contain substances that will help detoxify cells and keep them healthy. So, it' time to include healthy foods we may never have thought of adding to our pets' diets before.

You see, we all think of food in terms of carbohydrates, fats, and protein. The cell wall is made up of protein, and carbohydrates are used for energy. However, these basic food groups are unable to maintain the body's health.

Vitamins, minerals, and phytonutrients are the tools that detoxify, and they are much needed by the cells to repair themselves, thus keeping the organs healthy. Vitamins and minerals are involved in the chemical processes that occur in cells every minute of every day.

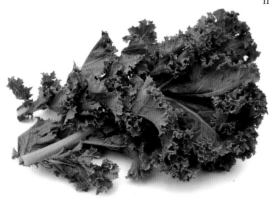

The beautiful colors in fruits and vegetables are created from phytonutrients. Certain fruits and vegetables, because of their powerful disease preventing effects, have been dubbed superfoods. In 1992, Johns Hopkins Medical School found the first phytonutrients in kale. While vitamins' effects last for a few hours, phytonutrients last for days, dumping toxins and promoting health.

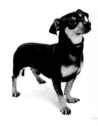
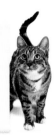

Chlorophyll is a super-healthy nutrient. Dogs seem to inherently know that it's healthy for them because they eat grass. Unfortunately, grass is grown to create a lawn rather than to be healthy for pets. Grass can't be digested. A dog may have the right idea when he eats grass, but the sad truth is that he does this because he has no other source of chlorophyll. In the wild, carnivores get their chlorophyll from the intestines of their prey. They also have a plethora of healthy wild plants to nibble on.

Chlorophyll helps to cleanse all of the body's cells, fight infection, heal wounds, build the immune system, and detoxify all systems, particularly the liver and the digestive system. It also promotes digestive health, which is also why many dogs with digestive problems tend to go for the grass.

Our pet's livers are very important organs. The liver is the body's main detoxifier of chemicals, poisons, and toxins. Unfortunately, in today's world, our pets carry a heavy toxic load, and their livers, along with their kidneys, are tasked with the job of eliminating these toxins as best as they can. Chronic health problems can often result from a toxic load, so we need to do what we can to help our pets detox.

And that's particularly important in the springtime. *Why particularly in the springtime?* you might ask. Interestingly enough, in the spring, the pineal gland is stimulated by the increase in available natural light. As a result, the pineal gland stimulates the body to naturally detox. (That's why horses eat strange and seemingly unpalatable greenery in the springtime.) Think of it as the body's spring cleaning!

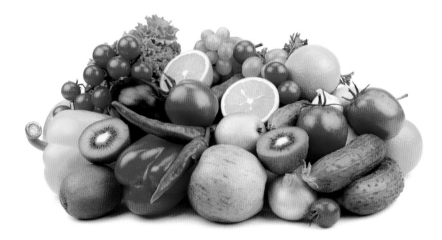

The Best Weed in Town—Dandelion Detox

Many gardeners consider dandelions a weed to be eliminated from the yard, but dandelions have many valuable properties, so you may want to stop and reconsider before you yank them out of the ground.

It's wonderful that the planet provides us with the tools we need for a natural spring cleaning of the body. Dandelions are one of these tools. They're abundant in the spring—exactly when we want to do a detox. Dandelions—as long as they are not treated with lawn chemicals—are super-healthy for detoxing. In fact, dandelion is one of my favorite herbs.

Dandelion is a more powerful liver tonic than milk thistle. Milk thistle protects the liver from damage, but dandelion can detoxify, protect, and heal the liver. It also flushes the kidneys. Additionally, dandelion moves toxins through and out of the lymphatic system.

The dandelion's roots sink deep into history. The plant has been around for thirty million years, as evidenced by dandelion fossils! Dandelion was well known in ancient times and was used in Egyptian, Greek, and Chinese cultures for just about every ailment. In the Middle Ages, almost every monastery had a physic garden—an herb garden with medicinal plants, which contained the herbs they needed for cooking and healing. The powerfully healing dandelion plant was certainly one of them.

Before the days of lawns, the dandelion's leaves and flowers were praised as a bounty of medicine. Gardeners would actually weed out the grass to make room for the dandelions. Dandelions were also world-famous for their beauty and cherished as decorative plants. They were beloved garden flowers in Europe and in the New World, a sweet reminder of home. In Japan, horticultural societies developed exciting new varieties for gardeners. Today, dandelions are sprayed with herbicides and considered unwanted guests. Only in the twentieth century have humans decided that the dandelion is a weed.

Dandelions are actually good for your lawn. Their wide-spreading roots loosen hard-packed soil, aerate the earth, and help reduce erosion while their deep taproots pull nutrients, such as calcium, from deep in the soil, making them available to other plants. Dandelions fertilize the grass. They are resistant to diseases, bugs, heat, cold, wind, rain, and human beings. To this day, herbalists hail the dandelion as the perfect plant medicine.

Dandelion tonics have been used and are still used to clean and tone the liver and remove toxins from the bloodstream. Dandelion reduces congestion in the liver and can even help with jaundice. Both the roots and the leaves can be used for medicinal purposes. The leaves work as a digestive and liver tonic as well as to flush and tone the kidneys, while the roots are used as a cleansing tonic for gallstones, jaundice, and constipation. Dandelions have been used successfully for dandruff, toothaches, sores, fevers, and rotting gums.

Dandelion is a wonderful example of how a complete herb works. It is a very powerful diuretic and is also one of the best sources of potassium. While pharmaceutical diuretics drain potassium out of the body and deplete potassium reserves, the dandelion root works to both remove excess fluid from the body and replace potassium that is lost in the process.

Dandelions are more nutritious than most of the vegetables in your garden. You can enjoy a complete meal, from salad greens to dandelion wine. If you overindulge, a cup of dandelion tea is the perfect remedy to help the liver flush hangover-inducing toxins from the body. And in the morning, you can have a coffee substitute made from toasted, ground dandelion roots.

So the next time a young child brings you a bouquet of dandelions as a special gift, just pretend you are living a few hundred years ago, and the flowers will seem as precious to you as they do to him or her.

To make dandelion tea:

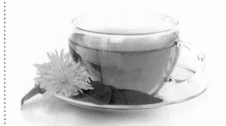

Place two to three tablespoons of dandelion leaves into one cup of water and bring to a boil. Simmer gently for fifteen minutes and let cool.

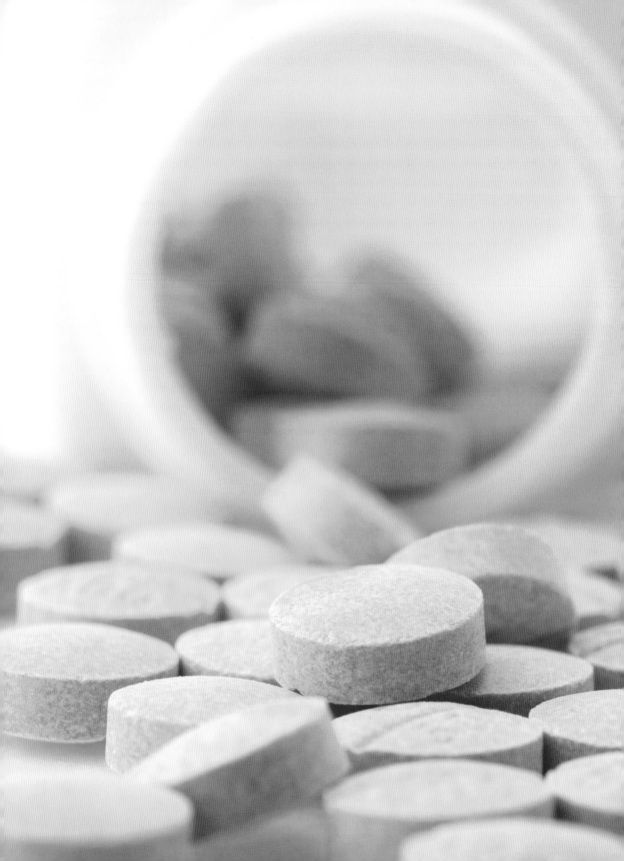

Chapter 9

Drug Dependence and Dangers: Their Inner Workings

Pharmaceutical drugs work differently from holistic products: they typically alleviate symptoms, but they rarely cure. At best, pharmaceuticals buy time while the body heals; at worst, they destroy the biological machinery in the body that our pets need to stay healthy and avoid diseases like cancer. Taking a painkiller for a headache stops the pain while the body works to heal itself. Someone suffering from migraine headaches truly appreciates the relief, but the drug does not correct the actual problem or make the body stronger. In all too many cases, the illness becomes chronic because the real source of the problem has not been found and corrected.

Simply treating a symptom curtails the body's ability to completely heal. The holistic approach assumes that the body is intelligent and that the symptoms are there for a reason. This is not to say that you should leave an illness or disease untreated, or that you should assume that your pet will heal on his or her own. Holistic treatments can be powerful tools that complement and enforce the body's innate ability to rebalance and restore itself, thus allowing the body to overcome the disease. Too many of us have long forgotten that the innate wisdom in the body, along with a little help from some holistic friends, can recreate true health.

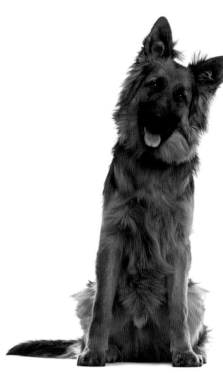

Typically, people with chronic problems refill their pharmaceutical prescriptions over and over again, month after month. Patients depend on their medications, which is very good for the pharmaceutical companies' bottom line. Dispensing a pill that would actually cure your high blood pressure or arthritis permanently would be very bad for business.

Winning the Battle and Losing the War

Remember, the modus operandi of pharmaceutical drugs is to eliminate symptoms. But it's the symptoms of an illness that alert you to the fact that something is wrong. When you feel your child's forehead and discover that he or she has a fever, that symptom is telling you something. In fact, the fever is making your child's body an inhospitable place for certain bacteria or a virus. The conventional drug aspirin will reduce the fever, but it has been proven to significantly lengthen recovery time. Echinacea, a holistic product made from the common coneflower, will work to break the fever quickly while supporting the immune system.

The dashboard of your automobile is equipped with a system of signals, or "symptoms." When the oil light goes on, it is a symptom that shows you that your engine needs oil. You could quickly suppress that symptom by finding the fuse box and pulling out the fuse that feeds your dashboard. The light is off, so everything is just fine. Or is it? We can blissfully forget that we have a problem—until it is too late—but we all know that this car will soon suffer significant engine damage because of the lack of oil.

In our pets' bodies, suppressing symptoms means impairing important biological mechanisms, only to result in severe diseases later on. That's the problem we're seeing with some of the allergy medications on the market. For many years, veterinarians prescribed steroids such as prednisone, prednisolone, and dexamethasone to reduce the allergic symptoms in our pets. Cortisol is a natural compound produced by the adrenal gland. Too much cortisol from external sources, in the form of these medications, suppresses the body's immune system.

You know by now that allergies and intolerances result from the immune system "misbehaving," so bringing that immune system to its knees may give the appearance of fixing the problem, but it really doesn't. In fact, when your pet stops taking the steroid medication, the problem comes right back. Steroids don't solve any medical problems, and veterinarians know that they only mask the symptoms of allergies. Plus, our pets really need their immune systems, especially with the epidemic incidence of cancer nowadays. The use of steroids seems to be declining as veterinarians are moving to more powerfully suppressive drugs for the immune system.

Cyclosporine

Consider Buffy's story: Nothing seemed to be helping Buffy, an affectionate buff-colored Cocker Spaniel. His owner was interested in holistic avenues. She brought Buffy to a veterinary dermatologist after she had tried everything, even steroids, and nothing had helped. The dermatologist prescribed cyclosporine for Buffy, and the improvement was almost immediate. Buffy's owner couldn't understand why her regular veterinarian (who was aware of the owner's holistic bent) and her holistic veterinarian had not prescribed cyclosporine previously.

The truth is that many veterinarians, both holistic and conventional, shudder when they contemplate this drug. One of my clients—a nurse—contacted me after her veterinarian had suggested cyclosporine. She explained to me the strict rules and precautions that she needed to take when administering it to human patients, which made her very wary of using the product on her dog.

Why does cyclosporine seem to be effective in cases where steroids don't work? What does it do? How does it work? What are the risks?

Cyclosporine is a mycotoxin. Mycotoxins are harmful products produced by fungi. Mycotoxins are chemical in nature, and they suppress immune function. Fungi rely on the mycotoxins they produce to kill any bacteria, other fungi, viruses, and anything else that might compete with them. Some examples of mycotoxins found in nature are aflatoxins (the most potent carcinogen on earth) and ochratoxins, which are both produced by *Aspergillus* fungi. Medical mycotoxins include a chemotherapy drug and a cholesterol-lowering drug.

The immunosuppressive effects of cyclosporine were discovered in Switzerland in 1972, and the drug was used successfully in preventing organ rejection in kidney transplants and later in liver transplants. In a transplant patient, it suppresses the immune system so the person's body does not reject its transplanted organ. Apart from transplant medicine, cyclosporine is used for a variety of skin conditions in both humans and pets.

The side effects of this drug include headaches, nausea, vomiting, diarrhea, hand tremors, swollen or bleeding gums, cancer, kidney failure, hypertension, easy bruising, hearing problems, yellowing of skin and eyes, loss of consciousness, vision changes, swollen glands, and dizziness. However, it's interesting to note that these aren't actually "side effects" at all, but rather symptoms of poisoning caused by this mycotoxin. Farmers are familiar with the deleterious effects experienced by animals that eat moldy grain containing mycotoxins, and the symptoms all agree. In fact, death is one side effect listed on the feline prescription.

The literature on cyclosporine prescribed for people states that their risk of infection will be higher while they are taking this drug. Patients are warned to avoid people with contagious diseases or infections. Of course, your pets will have the same increased risk for infection and cancer. Owners are instructed to wash their hands after applying cyclosporine to their dogs or cats. Heck, I'd suit up and wear latex gloves if I ever had to apply the product.

Here's another interesting tidbit. I had a client who worked in the laboratories of a prestigious pharmaceutical company, doing tests to determine the side effects of many different drugs. She told me that they did initial testing protocols to set up the study and observed when the side effects occur. Let's say, for example, that after ninety days, 40 percent of the rats developed cancer and 20 percent went into liver failure. The company would then use this information to design a study that lasts for no more than sixty or seventy days so that the study ended before any side effects happened. They could then state that they found side effects in only a very tiny percentage of the studied cases.

It took many years of practicing medicine for me to fully understand that drug companies want to make money and not cure illnesses. If one pill would cure your high blood pressure, what would happen to the pharmaceutical company's monthly revenue if you stopped going in for refills? Similarly, no pet vaccination company brags that its vaccinations last for ten or more years because of the revenue that they would lose due to the decrease in annual vaccinations.

A Collie owner once called me in distress. After being on cyclosporine for a month or two, her dog had developed fast-growing masses on the upper and lower gums. They couldn't surgically remove them fast enough. Of course, the veterinary oncologist immediately took the dog off of the cyclosporine. In fact, every oncologist immediately takes any pet off of this drug.

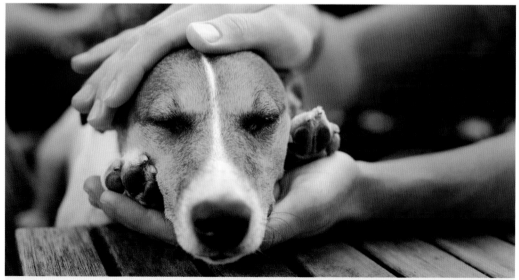

Your pet's health and well-being lie in your hands.

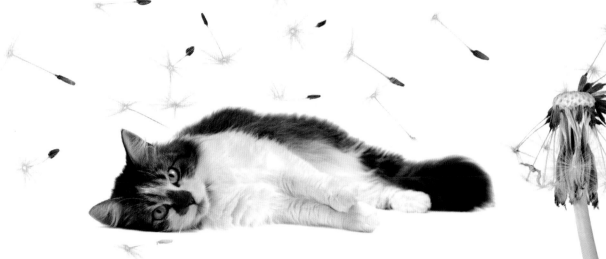

Veterinarians who care and who also understand the mechanism behind how cyclosporine works shiver in their shoes. They wouldn't use it on their dogs and cats, and you shouldn't use it on yours. For many of my veterinary friends, the mere mention of this product renders us at a loss for words.

As pet owners began researching cyclosporine, they became leery about using it on their best friends. At the same time, the pharmaceutical industry was busy coming up with yet another set of compounds that would obliterate our pets' immune systems.

Oclacitinib

If your pet is on oclacitinib, read this section and stop administering the drug as soon as you can. Here, you're going to find out how it demolishes essential parts of your pet's internal disease-fighting systems. This is another drug that veterinary oncologists immediately discontinue. Let me tell you about it.

Kinases are important messenger/signaling compounds that the body's cells use to communicate with each other. Kinases are very important because they are totally responsible for the function of and communication between many diverse systems in our pets' bodies. An Australian chemist happened to discover some new kinases, which are known as JAK1, JAK2, JAK3, and TKY2.

These particular kinases are key elements in controlling both growth and development, and they do the following work:

- Police the body against tumor formation
- Control the body's growth and development
- Form white and red blood cells
- Provide immunity with proper functioning of your pets antibody-producing cells (B-cells) and "policing" cells (T-cells)
- Control inflammation

It was the 1980s when pharmaceutical companies saw the opportunity to create a drug that would stop these JAKs in their tracks. They sure succeeded.

Oclacitinib interrupts and stops the Janus kinases from working, and your pet cannot live healthfully without their functions. For example, your pet's antibody system (B-cells) and killer-cell

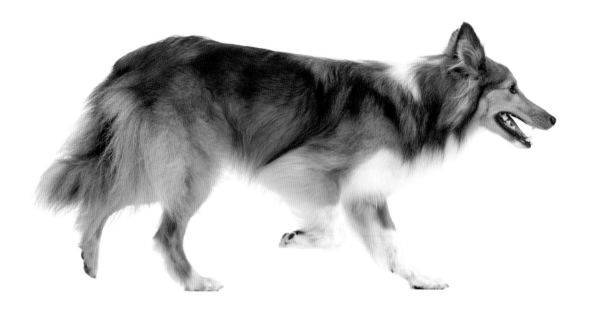

system (T-cells) require the presence of JAK3. JAK1 is vital for the constant surveillance within your pet's body to find and destroy abnormal cells that have become cancerous before they form tumors. JAK1 also is an imperative messenger necessary for destroying invasive parasites, fungi, bacteria, and viruses. JAK2 is central to the production of bone-marrow stem cells, which become red and white blood cells and platelets. All of these JAKs talk to each other and share information to maintain health in your pet's body.

Sometimes I feel that the world of modern medicine has gone mad. One in two dogs is getting cancer. Cancer in cats is on the rise. We all know this. In the wake of this knowledge, a new anti-itch drug comes along and opens the door wide to cancer with a welcome sign on it to boot. Oclacitinib (which few may have understood until reading this information), stops that worrisome and, at times, intolerable itching with the repercussions of cancer, low white cell count, low red cell count, stunted growth, and more. If your pet is currently taking this drug, reread the warnings and side effects, and they'll make more sense to you this time.

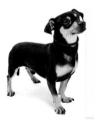

Did You Know?

JAK initially stood for "just another kinase," but these kinases are now officially known as *Janus* kinases, named for the two-faced Roman god of the same name.

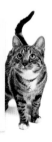

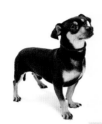
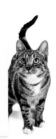
Monoclonal Antibody Therapy

Monoclonal antibody therapy (mAb) is a therapy specifically for dogs and tailor-made to be accepted by only a dog's immune system. It is given as an injection that usually begins to work immediately and continues to work for four to five weeks. It supposedly inhibits the nerve response of itch to immune stimulation. Because it is actually a dog antibody, it's not technically considered a drug.

The term *moloclonal* means that the antibodies are targeted to one protein—this is the protein that causes the dog to itch, and it is believed to have no other function in the body. This therapy is intended to neutralize the itch-causing protein before it starts the itch. It was designed to go after just one messenger molecule—IL-31—not a whole class of messenger molecules like oclacitinib does. Every kinase communicates with others in a cascading effect. Inhibiting one kinase affects hundreds of other kinases.

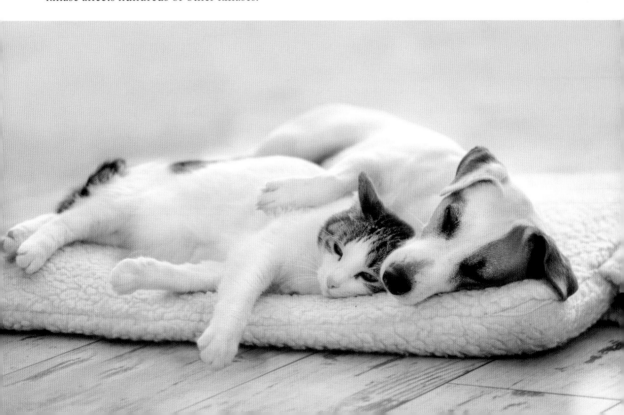

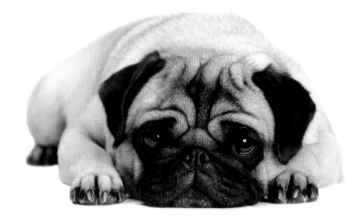

No one completely understands how this therapy really works. At the time of writing, the pharmaceutical companies are still quite early into the learning experience and studies. Some material suggests that mAb decreases the skin inflammation that causes itching, while other information suggests that it primarily blocks the nerve transmission of itch signals from the pet's skin to the brain. Some data states that the therapy effects both of these results.

We know little about what IL-31's normal roles in your dog's body are. But medical research does show and doctors do know that messenger chemicals in the IL-31 family are used *in different parts of the body for different purposes*. We know that some of IL-31's functions change, depending on the animal's stage of development and age. IL-31 receptors exist in many types of tissue throughout your dog's body, so IL-31 could in no way be restricted to just the "itching" functions in your pet's body.

Sensory nerves are receptive to IL-31, and your dog's skin cells receive IL-31 messages as well. So does the lining of your pet's lungs and muscle cells. We know that certain types of white cells along with other cells involved in the body's defenses receive IL-31 messages, too. IL-31 is also present in your dog's thymus gland, testes, spleen, and kidneys. When a drug destroys the IL-31 messages, cells with the IL-31 receptor are going to be affected—we just don't know exactly how.

Holistic Options

There are holistic treatments that are alternatives to these conventional drugs and that can cure dogs and cats. Because the animals are actually cured, they won't require constant diet changes and medications throughout the rest of their lives.

Additionally, these little IL-31 receptors receive and are activated by a second type of message from another signaling compound called oncostatin M (OSM), whose normal functions are just as poorly understood and complex as those of IL-31. It is known, though, that OSM's presence at normal levels is *critical* to good health.

Monoclonal antibody therapy is a journey into the unknown. Like the other treatments mentioned, mAb is not a cure, but an immune suppressor that must be administered over and over again. Years may pass before we know all the consequences of the use of this drug. When pharmaceutical companies enter the terrain of annihilating the essential messenger systems of the body they are entering dangerous territory in regards to our pet's health.

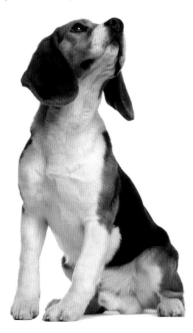

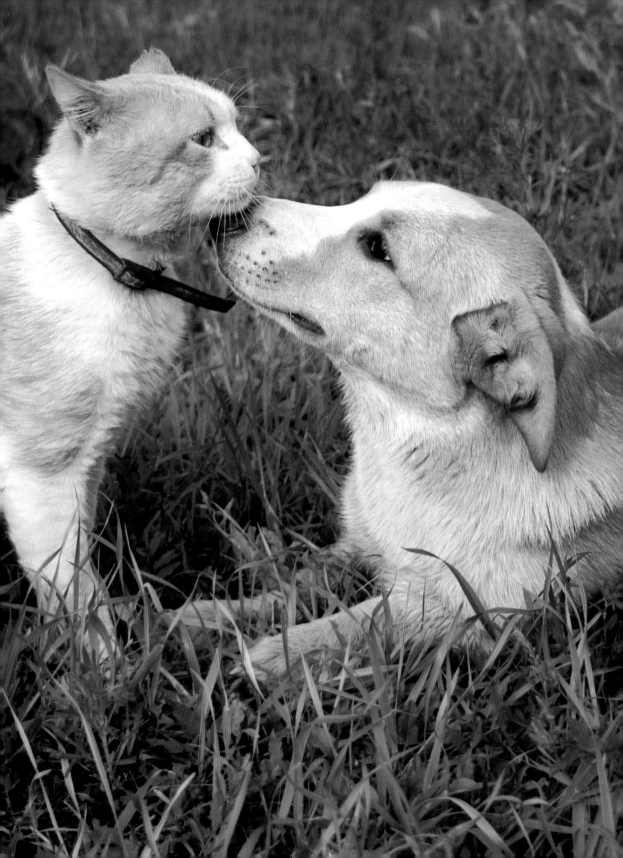

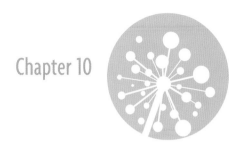

Allergy Impersonators: More Common than You Think

Before we discuss the best holistic treatment for your pet, we want you to be sure that an allergy or sensitivity or intolerance is the real culprit. Allergy impersonators can look like allergies, act like allergies, and smell like allergies.

Impersonating the "Itchies"

We all tend to think that a diagnosed allergy is only and always a simple case of an allergic pet or one with food sensitivities. It's important to know that an allergic presentation may be accompanied by another problem that will intensify the itching. Any pet can develop secondary bacterial, fungal/yeast, or even mixed infections on his or her body, perhaps along with concurrent ear infections. If so, the secondary problem will need to be handled in addition to the allergic problem. That's because both may be causing itching.

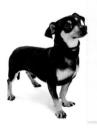

Did You Know?

Other factors that cause itching can occur independently of allergies. They can also occur concurrently with allergies. We must acknowledge and address these factors if we are to truly resolve our pet's problem.

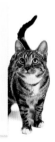

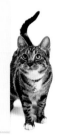

Copycat #1: Malassezia

Malassezia is a type of yeast. It lives on our pets' skin normally, but certain factors can cause it to overgrow, creating an infection and/or exacerbating other skin conditions. A malassezia infection all by itself is very itchy and will appear *just like an allergy*. In other cases, an allergy will cause skin inflammation, which will make the skin irritated and moist, resulting in yeast overgrowth. To top this off, some dogs start to have allergic reactions to the malassezia itself. It's a vicious cycle.

In dogs, this particular yeast loves to grow in moist areas, such as the folds of the toes, the underarms, the neck folds, and the belly area. Affected cats usually experience malassezia overgrowth in their ears, but the infection isn't nearly as common in cats as it is in dogs.

Malassezia occurs when the organism *Malassezia pachydermatis*, which is normal in small amounts on the skin and in the ear canal, overgrows and causes itching and inflammation of the skin. An infected dog may have a musty smell, or you will find a brown, slightly sweet-smelling substance in your dog's or cat's ears.

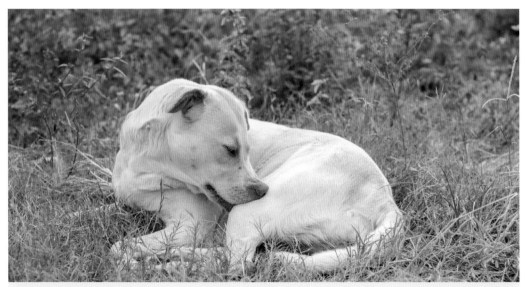

Skin problems and itchiness don't automatically point to allergies.

The Microbiome

Many different types of bacteria, along with yeast, are naturally present on our pets' skin. It's called the microbiome and is the first line of defense against infection. These different microbes live in a balanced state, respecting each other's boundaries. When one type of microbe, such as malassezia, steps over the line, so to speak, it grows out of control, usually causing intense itching for the animal.

Malassezia is commonly found on the thickened, denuded areas of the skin of dogs with chronic allergies, often in areas that sunlight cannot reach, such as the belly, lower neck, and underarms. The affected skin may look like someone sprinkled pepper on it, have little red bumps, and/or be flaky or crusty. When it occurs in the ears, you may find thickened, red ear flaps; itchy ears; and brown ear secretions. But it does not have to be this obvious. Malassezia can manifest in small ways, such as reddened skin in between the toes, or some brown crud at the top border of the toenail, or a dark grayish patch on the skin.

The allergy and the yeast infection play off of each other, each one contributing to the other's ability to cause a problem. The allergy makes it easier for the yeast to take hold, and its presence makes the itching worse, sometimes causing the skin to become thickened and dark.

It's important to know if your dog has malassezia in addition to allergies because the malassezia will cause the itching to persist even after the allergies begin to improve. That's why I recommend that you treat the yeast infection, if present, concurrently.

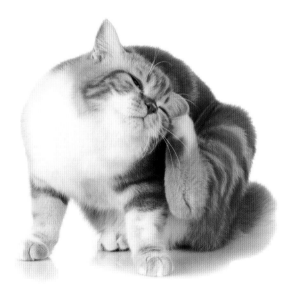

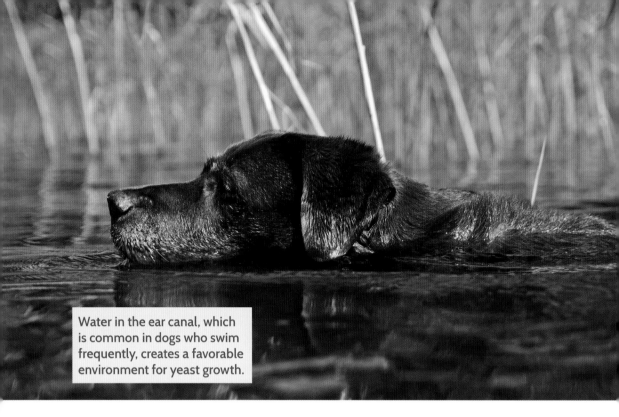

Water in the ear canal, which is common in dogs who swim frequently, creates a favorable environment for yeast growth.

I prefer a topical treatment for malassezia. There's a reason for this—please indulge me in a personal story: I had an area on my lower neck that I self-diagnosed as malassezia, so I began taking what is considered the best antifungal for malassezia—ketoconazole—according to the directions. After taking the medication twice a day for two weeks with no results, I went to the dermatologist, thinking that my diagnosis was incorrect. The dermatologist told me that I had the right diagnosis. He then told me that I should take one pill, eat a little food, and then go to the gym an hour later and work out until I was really sweating. I did what he told me, and it worked.

Here's the rub: dogs and cats don't sweat the way that we do, so we have to go with topical treatment for malassezia. Malassezia infection often begins with an ear infection from the yeast (we'll discuss ear infections later in the book, as they play a role in many cases of allergies), but it can occur on its own and/or result from localized inflammation caused by allergies and intolerances.

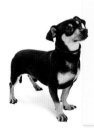

Did You Know?

While the bacterial infections of the skin are typically recognized and treated, fungal and yeast infections can often go undetected, resulting in frustration.

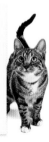

The treatments I like best for malassezia are those that contain natural, nontoxic enzymes that kill both yeast and bacteria. There is an enzymatic medicated shampoo that you can use on the affected areas, and an enzymatic medicated creme rinse that you apply to and leave on the affected areas. There is also a topical spray with a small concentration of hydrocortisone that you can use, in a pinch, when an area suddenly becomes very itchy. Additionally, enzymatic ear medications are great for the yeast infections that dogs, and occasionally cats, get in their ears.

Malassezia grows slowly yet tenaciously. It can be difficult to eradicate because once it is established, it is slow to recede. You have to persist over time with the enzymatic treatment.

Copycat #2: Scabies

Just like allergies, sarcoptic mange, or scabies, has also reached epidemic proportions in dogs. Sarcoptic mange in felines is uncommon, but notoedric mange in cats is very similar to sarcoptic mange in dogs and is often called "feline scabies." The beginning stages of scabies look just like a skin allergy or sensitivity. Pets with scabies, when cared for by doting owners, don't progress to the more advanced, and easy to detect, signs of scabies.

Scabies mites, resembling microscopic crabs, tunnel deep into the animal's skin, causing localized reactions and irritation. Because they live deep in the skin, and superficial skin scrapings usually produce negative results, veterinarians often advise treating the pet for scabies, which is safe and

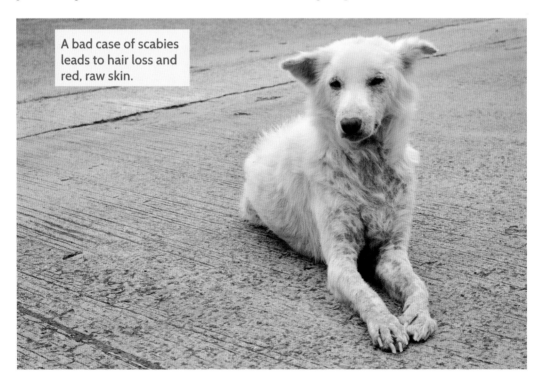

A bad case of scabies leads to hair loss and red, raw skin.

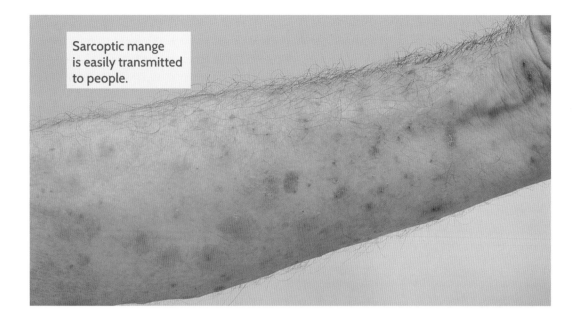

Sarcoptic mange is easily transmitted to people.

inexpensive, before making an official diagnosis. You have the option of multiple skin biopsies under anesthesia, but the biopsies may or may not show the presence of mites, even in affected animals. That's the problem with this type of mange, and that's why it's often just easier to treat the pet for mange and see if there is an improvement. Therefore, if your pet suddenly starts to experience intense itching, it may be a good idea to treat for scabies before considering a diagnosis of allergies.

Scabies is very contagious and travels easily from pet to pet (think boarding kennels, groomers, dog parks). Foxes can also carry sarcoptic mange mites and transmit it to dogs. When the mites jump on people, they can cause red, itchy bumps in clusters on the skin. So if you happen to be getting small clusters of itchy bumps on your body at the same time your pet starts with ferocious itching, it's a good indication that you may be dealing with scabies.

A client named Anne used to bring her Cocker Spaniel, Holly, to me when I had my practice in Pennsylvania. She contacted me by phone when I was in New Zealand because her dog had been itching furiously for two years. Holly slept in Anne's bed, so Anne was also very itchy, with little red bumps on her skin. I was sure it was scabies. Her veterinarian, after two years of repeated visits, had referred her to a dermatologist. He was upset when she called me instead and was affronted that I presumed to diagnose scabies from across the world. Anne insisted on treating Holly for scabies, and it solved both of their problems.

One question I pose when considering scabies is the timing of the itching. Most of the time, allergic pets itch when they are lying around, doing pretty much nothing. Pets with scabies, however, stop cold in their tracks when playing, chasing, or eating a meal that they love to sit down and scratch away because the itchiness is so intense.

Signs and symptoms:

- Ferocious itching
- Pet stops to scratch when eating or playing
- Can look like a skin allergy
- Possibly other itchy pets in the household
- May have crusty area on tips of ears
- May notice itchy bumps on owner's skin

Your veterinarian will help you choose the best scabies treatment for your pet. If there is no response, your pet may not have scabies, and your veterinarian may start looking at allergies as the culprit.

Copycat #3: Ringworm

Ringworm occurs in both dogs and cats—perhaps even more so in cats. It's not actually a worm, despite its name, but a microscopic parasitic fungus that lives in the hair follicles. It's a hardy fungus that is present in the soil and on other surfaces; the spores can persist in the environment for up to two years. Cats can contract ringworm when they're exposed to infected soil and through contact with other cats; the same is true for dogs. Athlete's food and jock itch are two types of ringworm that people can get, often from public places.

Pets less than one year old, whose immune systems are still developing, are most susceptible. Ringworm first shows as a small, scaly skin lesion, which causes itching and often, but not always,

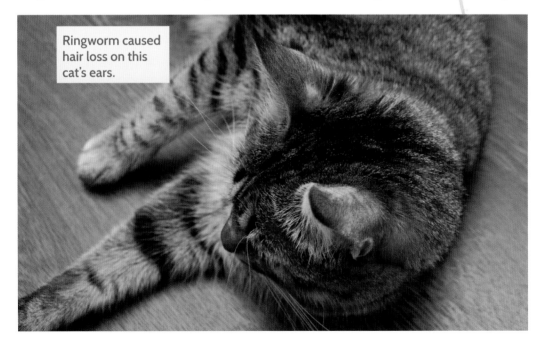

Ringworm caused hair loss on this cat's ears.

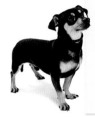

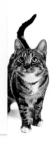

forms into a ring. Lesions usually appear on the underside of the body or other areas that do not get sun exposure. The pet may have a moth-eaten appearance to the fur, and secondary bacterial infections can occur within the circular area of fungus.

The appearance of this particular fungus dictates its name. A round area of fur is denuded as the fungus grows in a circular pattern. The far edge of the circle can have a red circular mark, and oftentimes the fur in the very middle of the circle is growing in, so the pattern appears as a ring. Ringworm can be easy to identify because of its appearance.

Copycat #4: Diarrhea from Parasites

There's a difference between acute diarrhea and the chronic diarrhea that often accompanies allergies and intolerances. And chronic diarrhea does not always signify an allergy or intolerance. Diarrhea from Parasites in dogs and cats can occur for a number of reasons.

By far, the most common cause of sudden, acute diarrhea is dietary indiscretion. A rapid change in diet or too many leftovers can cause sudden loose stool. I discuss natural solutions for acute diarrhea in Chapter 14. Because treatment for food allergies and intolerances can take some time,

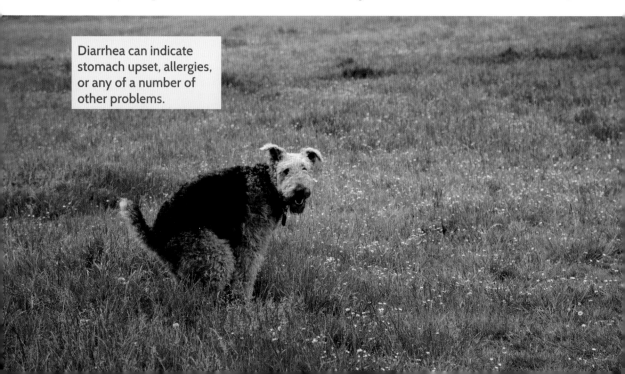

Diarrhea can indicate stomach upset, allergies, or any of a number of other problems.

these suggestions will be handy for anyone who has a pet with a chronic or acute gastrointestinal problem. Additionally, a viral infection, such as parvovirus in dogs or coronavirus in cats, can cause diarrhea, but these are far more rare than gastrointestinal causes.

Just as with itchy allergies, there are more common and simpler reasons for chronic diarrhea, and it's important to know how to identify and treat them. Parasites and infections in the gut can cause chronic diarrhea, vomiting, and weight loss, and both cats and dogs can get a number of intestinal parasites and intestinal infections. The most common parasites are intestinal worms, for which the treatment is very easy. If your pet responds to deworming treatment, you may be able to rule out an allergy or intolerance.

We also need to include bugs like *Giardia*, *Clostridium*, and *Cryptosporidium* as important causes of diarrhea in dogs and cats. *Tritrichomonas foetus* can also cause diarrhea in cats.

The first step many of us take when confronted by diarrhea is to bring a stool sample to your veterinarian to test for worms. That's smart, because it's very easy for dogs and cats who go outside to get worms. We are relieved when the sample comes back "negative," meaning that no worm eggs were found in the pet's stool. However, a negative fecal test does not mean that your dog or cat does not have worms; it simply means that no worm eggs were found in the sample.

It's important for you to understand just how this works. I'll tell you a true story: At the University of Pennsylvania School of Veterinary Medicine, it was not uncommon for us to see dogs and cats with chronic diarrhea. Because the owners were bringing their pets to a renowned teaching facility, they were not averse to doing fecal test after fecal test to check and recheck over and over for worms if their pets had diarrhea.

I remember one case of unresolved diarrhea in a young dog where we did at least ten fecal exams, about once a week with each visit. Each one came back negative, meaning that we saw no worm eggs when viewing the sample under a microscope. Weren't we surprised when the owner came in with a plastic baggie of the roundworms that her dog had thrown up—after all those negative fecal tests.

Let's look at it this way: I have chickens. If I go to collect their eggs and find some, I should be able to deduce that there are chickens present who have laid eggs in my henhouse. If one day I find no eggs, I can't truthfully say that I have no chickens. They could have found an out-of-the-way place to deposit their eggs, or they could be having an off day.

Did You Know?

It's very common for a pet owner to bring in runny diarrhea for the stool sample when his or her dog or cat has diarrhea. The diarrhea dilutes the stool sample and makes the eggs of intestinal parasites even harder to find.

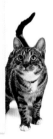

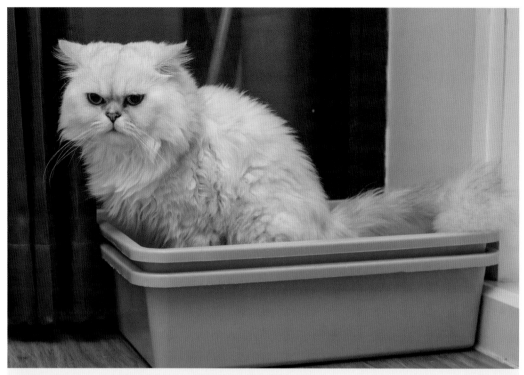

Keep an eye on your cat's litter box for any abnormalities.

Types of Worms and Bugs

Some of the common worms whose eggs can be found in a pet's stool are hookworms, roundworms, threadworms, and whipworms. Infection with the protozoa *Giardia* and *Coccidia* can also cause chronic diarrhea. Tapeworms are transmitted by fleas and do not produce eggs; rather, their segments break off and leave the body when they are ripe. These segments are found *on* the stool or around the anus but not *in* the stool.

Dogs can become infected with hookworms just by lying around at the dog park, watching the other dogs play. These parasites are called hookworms because they have hook-like mouthpieces that they use to attach themselves to the intestines. You see, a dog with hookworms relieves himself on the grass, and the eggs are transferred into the soil, where they develop into the larvae, which can survive for months before infecting your dog. These larvae can burrow right into your dog's skin as he plays or lies down in the grass.

If your dog drinks contaminated water in the park, or if he grooms his paws after spending time outdoors and some larvae have come aboard, he can become infected with hookworms. Cats often get hookworms when they groom their feet. Hookworms can also be ingested by a rat or mouse, and if your cat eats one of those little fellows, she can get hookworms. However, hookworms are much more common in dogs than cats.

Once hookworms have entered your pet's body, they travel through it like something out of *The X-Files*, winding up in the intestine. Without any GPS, they know just where to go. Once a pet gets hookworms, he or she can get not only diarrhea but also bloody stool and even anemia. Because the worms take a while to mature and shed eggs, initial fecal tests may show nothing.

Puppies and kittens are commonly born with roundworms. Female dogs and cats have encysted roundworm larvae in their body tissues. The hormones of pregnancy activate the larvae, which then migrate through the mother's tissues and end up right in the uterus, infecting the yet-to-be-born puppies or kittens. The mother's milk also transfers roundworm larvae to the nursing pups or kittens. In both cases, these parasites make it to the intestines of the youngsters to set up housekeeping. Because worming medications work only on intestinal worms, worming a female dog or cat before she becomes pregnant will have no effect on the larvae already encysted in the tissues.

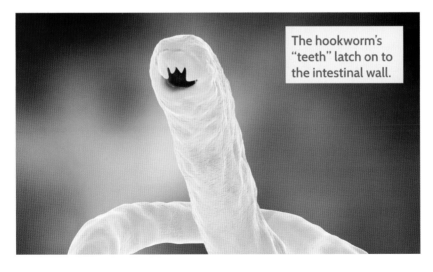

The hookworm's "teeth" latch on to the intestinal wall.

Female roundworms can produce 200,000 eggs in just one day. The eggs are protected by hard shells, so they can exist in the soil for years. When dogs or cats groom their feet or happen to ingest infected soil or stool, the roundworms get into their systems and make their way to the intestines.

Whipworms are seen more commonly in dogs than cats. This worm sheds comparatively few eggs; therefore, multiple stool samples may not reveal their presence. If a dog has chronic weight loss and passes stool that seems to have a covering of mucus (especially the last portion of the stool that the dog passes), he may be infected with whipworms. Once again, Panacur, containing fenbendazole, is available over the counter and is safe and easy to administer as a powder on the food for three days.

After reading about these different parasites, you may be ready to run to the heartworm preventives that have extras for treating intestinal worms or the flea and tick products that also promise protection from worms. I do not recommend that you do this. No pet needs so many toxins every month to protect against what a once-yearly worming with Panacur will accomplish. Remember, we're talking about minimizing toxic exposure.

Now you know how easy it is for your pet to get worms, and you understand that you can worm your pet if he or she experiences a diarrhea or GI problem, particularly if your pet is in situations where he or she is susceptible to picking up worms. I'm contacted often by people with pets who have diarrhea problems. You'd be amazed how many pet owners object when I suggest that we start with a simple worming treatment. "How could my pet get worms?" they ask. It's easier than you think…and now you know why.

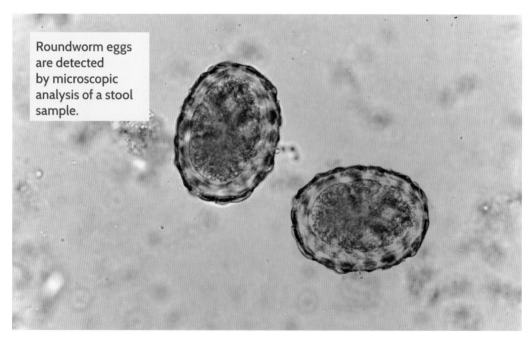

Roundworm eggs are detected by microscopic analysis of a stool sample.

Tapeworms

Tapeworms are common in both dogs and cats. Apparently, fleas think that tapeworm eggs are very tasty. Tapeworms are then transmitted to dogs and cats that ingest fleas. When you think of a cat grooming herself or a dog chewing away at an itch on his skin, you can understand how easy it is to ingest them. Another method of transmission is eating wildlife or rodents that have either tapeworms or fleas.

Tapeworms can reach 4 to 6 inches (10 to 15 cm) in length within the pet's intestine. Each worm may have as many as ninety segments, with the head at one end and many tiny brick-like repeating segments following. The segments farthest from the head detach. They come out in the stool and can be seen as little rice-sized pieces attached to the fur around the anal area. If you see what looks like dried rice on your cat's favorite cushion, you've got to consider tapeworms.

Because these worms break into segments and do not lay eggs, a fecal exam will not show anything worthwhile. Tapeworms are also not killed by the typical worming medications that are used for the other intestinal worms. Panacur will kill certain tapeworms but is not very effective against the common tapeworm. Drontal Plus contains praziquantel, which effectively kills tapeworms. Tapeworms have a tough cuticle covering that protects them against digestion, and this drug dissolves that cuticle.

In my practice, after treating with the recommended dose, owners would report that the tapeworms had returned. Because it was too soon for a new tapeworm to have developed and started to shed, I realized that the initial tapeworms had not been killed. You see, the heads of the tapeworms have thicker cuticles, which would protect them. That's why, with tapeworms, I usually treat first with an injection of Drontal® Plus and follow it up with the oral tablet about two weeks later. I like to feel secure that they're all dead and gone.

Intestinal Lymphoma

Lymphosarcoma, or lymphoma, is becoming more and more common in both dogs and cats. There are many different ways that this particular kind of cancer can manifest and many different organs or organ systems that it can invade. In our case, we're concerned about intestinal lymphoma because it can look just like IBD—so much so that it becomes difficult for the veterinarian and the radiologist to differentiate the two on an ultrasound because the ultrasound often shows thickened intestinal walls in both cases.

Intestinal lymphoma and IBD are both too common in cats. It's important to know that IBD and the chronic intestinal inflammation that it causes can predispose cats to intestinal lymphoma. In dogs, the more common presentation of lymphosarcoma is enlarged lymph nodes, but dogs can also get intestinal lymphoma.

Just like with IBD and some parasitic infections, lymphosarcoma causes diarrhea and weight loss, sometimes along with vomiting and a lack of appetite. Cats and dogs have the same symptoms, and cats can also have unkempt coats and be listless.

Because an ultrasound often cannot tell intestinal lymphoma and IBD apart, needle-guided aspirates are usually recommended. As with any aspirate, a representative sample is needed, but there is a chance that normal tissue will be aspirated instead of the cancerous area. The pathologist will always state that a nonrepresentative sample could have been obtained.

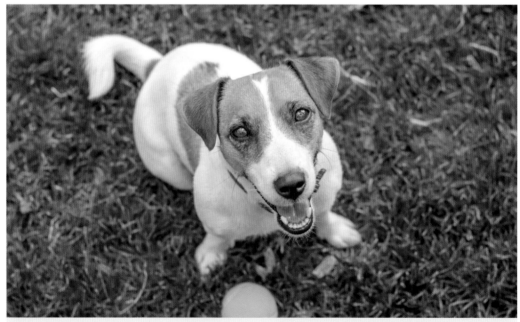

Whether allergies or cancer, early detection and treatment is always the best course of action.

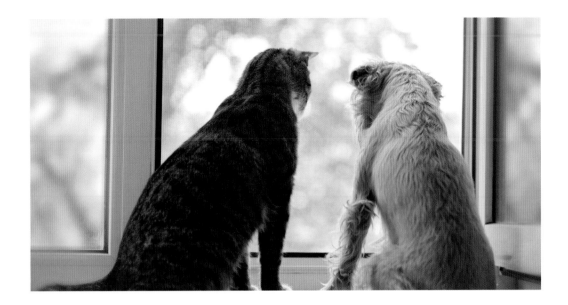

When lymphoma of the intestine is a possibility, you need accurate tests and good veterinary care. The Veterinary Diagnostics Institute (*http://vdilab.com*) has both a feline and a canine test available, and testing requires only drawing some blood and sending it to the laboratory. The TK Feline Cancer Panel and the TK Canine Cancer Panel are used to detect many different cancers, including the differential diagnosis of intestinal lymphoma versus IBD.

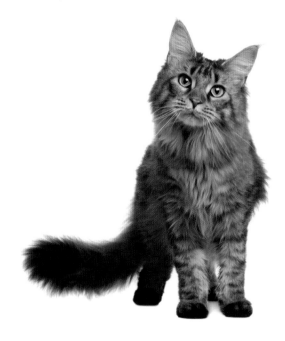

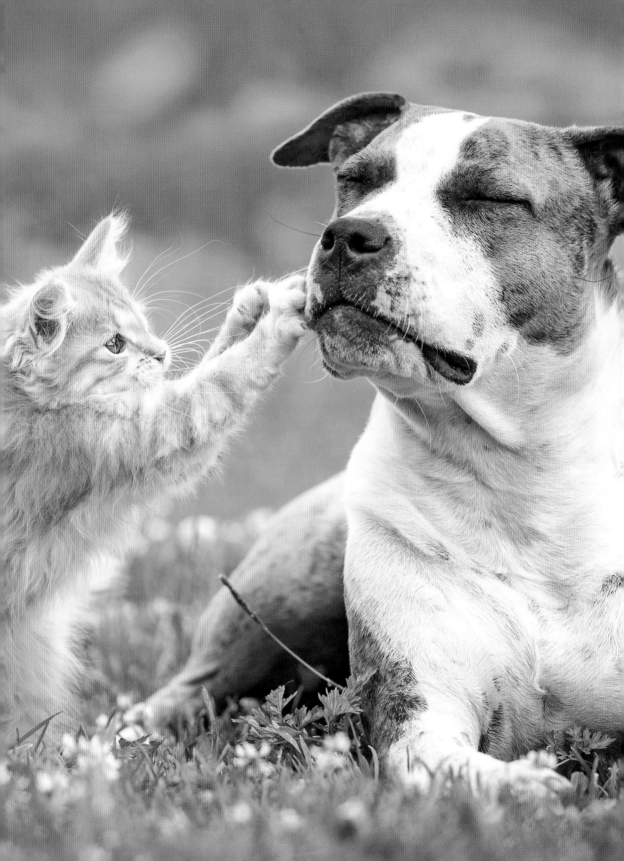

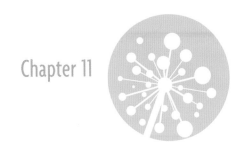

Chapter 11

Influential Organs and Glands: Thyroid, Liver, and More

Thinking Thyroid

Thyroid problems can contribute greatly to the allergic symptoms that animals exhibit. Checking your pet's thyroid requires a simple blood test that, at the minimum, tests the thyroid compounds T4 and free T4. These two readings will help determine if your pet's thyroid is underactive (hypothyroidism), which is fairly common in dogs but very rare in cats (cats are more likely to have overactive thyroid, or hyperthyroidism). If your veterinarian diagnoses hypothyroidism, he or she should prescribe supplemental thyroid medication.

Dogs younger than five years of age are not nearly as likely to be hypothyroid as older dogs. More than 70 percent of the close to 200 breeds recognized by the American Kennel Club consider hypothyroidism a major health concern. Just a few

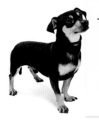

Did You Know?

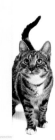

The thyroid is a very important master gland, and it regulates the performance of many important organs as well as the immune system. Often, after a pet's thyroid problem is corrected, allergies subside and secondary infections no longer occur because the immune system goes back to working correctly.

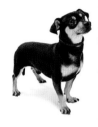
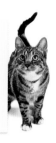

Did You Know?

Ingredients in flea and tick collars and in oral and spot-on flea and tick products have been proven irrefutably to be toxic and destructive to the thyroid gland.

of the many common breeds most affected, according to Michigan State University, are the Old English Sheepdog, Boxer, American Pit Bull Terrier, German Wirehaired Pointer, Maltese, Beagle, Dalmatian, Cocker Spaniel, Golden Retriever, Alaskan Malamute, Shetland Sheepdog, Irish Setter, Siberian Husky, Great Dane, Poodle, Labrador Retriever, Dachshund, and Doberman Pinscher.

I like to send bloodwork for thyroid tests to Dr. Jean Dodds' Hemopet laboratory in California because she has unquestionable expertise in the area of thyroid disease. She has an excellent test, Thyroid Panel 5, that tests for T4, free T4, T3, and free T3 along with autoantibodies. Getting a complete panel such as this leaves no stone unturned as far as thyroid function is concerned. Other veterinary laboratories, such as ANTECH (*www.antechdiagnostics.com*) and IDEXX (*www.idexx.com*), also do various combination tests for thyroid function.

Thyroid problems not only can contribute greatly to the allergic symptoms your pet exhibits but also can slow his or her response to any kind of therapy, whether holistic or conventional. Hypothyroidism in dogs can contribute to difficult-to-treat malassezia yeast problems. The thyroid has a very important role in immune-system function.

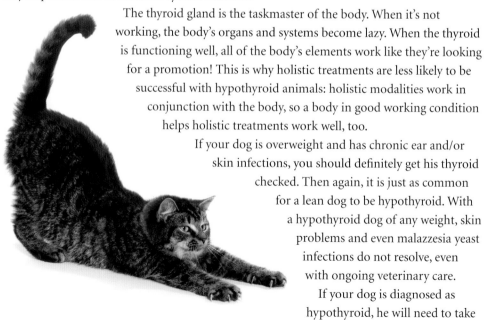

The thyroid gland is the taskmaster of the body. When it's not working, the body's organs and systems become lazy. When the thyroid is functioning well, all of the body's elements work like they're looking for a promotion! This is why holistic treatments are less likely to be successful with hypothyroid animals: holistic modalities work in conjunction with the body, so a body in good working condition helps holistic treatments work well, too.

If your dog is overweight and has chronic ear and/or skin infections, you should definitely get his thyroid checked. Then again, it is just as common for a lean dog to be hypothyroid. With a hypothyroid dog of any weight, skin problems and even malazzesia yeast infections do not resolve, even with ongoing veterinary care.

If your dog is diagnosed as hypothyroid, he will need to take

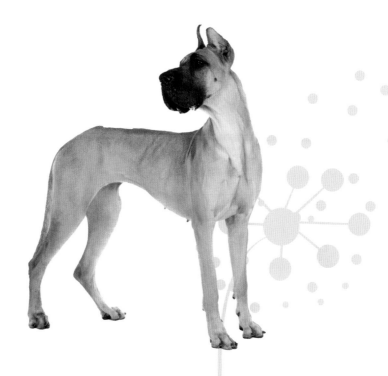

inexpensive thyroid medication twice a day. Humans usually take thyroid medication once a day, but dogs metabolize it much faster than we do, so always make sure that your vet gives you the twice-a-day dosage for your dog.

Loving the Liver

The liver plays an important role in digestion. Before the nutrients from food enter the bloodstream to be distributed around the body, they travel via the portal vein into the liver. The liver then monitors the contents of the blood and removes any toxic and poisonous substances before they can reach the rest of the body.

The liver has three main detoxification pathways:

1. Filtering the blood to remove large toxins;
2. Enzymatically breaking down unwanted chemicals and poisons, such as medications, pesticides, and enterotoxins from the intestines; and
3. Making bile, which is used, in part, to excrete fat-soluble toxins and poisons.

Blood detoxification is critical because blood is loaded with bacteria, endotoxins, antigen–antibody complexes, and other toxic substances. A healthy liver clears almost 100 percent of bacteria and other toxins from the blood before the blood enters general circulation.

As we discussed earlier in the book, our pets are inundated with toxins every single day: flea and tick products, herbicides, lawn chemicals, and the list goes on. To put it mildly, our dogs' and cats' livers are overloaded in today's world. This kind of toxic load doesn't necessarily show up in a blood test. Inflammation of the liver is indicated by elevated liver enzymes, but we're talking about the liver's job of handling toxins.

The Antioxidant That Rules Them All: Glutathione

Glutathione exists in every cell. It protects the cells' tiny but important engines, the mitochondria. This little protein made up of three amino acids is the king of all antioxidants in the body. Without gluthathione, cells would simply disintegrate and die from unrestrained oxidation. Our more familiar antioxidants, such as vitamins C and E, have short life spans, but glutathione has the ability to bring back spent antioxidants from the dead and even recharge itself.

Because all other antioxidants depend on glutathione to function properly, and because glutathione is the most important, abundant, active, and powerful of the antioxidants, doctors call it the master antioxidant. None of the over-the-counter antioxidants would work without the glutathione created in the cells. The highest levels of glutathione exist in the liver, and it's no accident that the liver is the major organ of detoxification. The liver desperately needs its glutathione to stay healthy and to complete its detoxification process.

When I need to support a dog or cat with a liver problem, I prescribe transdermal glutathione or injectable glutathione through a compounding pharmacy. (By the way, glutathione works incredibly well in patients with kidney problems, especially cats.)

Protecting Health with pH

During the days of the dinosaurs, the oxygen content of the earth's atmosphere was 50 percent. Scientists actually took tiny bubbles found in arctic ice and amber and removed the air in them

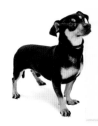
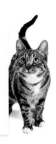

to measure their oxygen content. In the early twentieth century, the oxygen content of the atmosphere was 38 percent. In the twenty-first century, it's around 21 percent.

We all breathe oxygen. When oxygen levels are high, the red blood cells pick up the extra oxygen and provide it to the cells and tissues. More oxygen means more efficient waste and toxin removal. Cells function better when they have ample oxygen available to them. Importantly, most disease-producing organisms, as well as cancer, like environments with little or no oxygen.

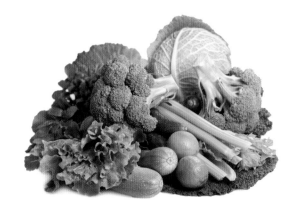

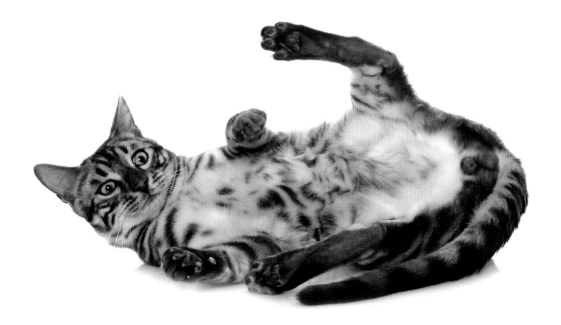

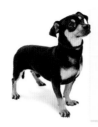
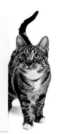

Did You Know?

The liver can process forty times more toxins than the kidneys, and it functions forty times better in an alkaline environment. That all adds up.

Oxygen also helps neutralize the acids in our body, such as the lactic acid that results from muscle overload. Oxygenated cells burn fat more efficiently. Ample oxygen assists in the digestion of foods and creates energy. Because all the cells in your dog's body perform better when they have enough oxygen, immune system function also improves.

Our dogs and cats are living in a very different world from that of the dinosaurs. Dinosaurs could never be considered "couch potatoes." While some moved quickly and some more slowly, they all moved. They all had to search for food and water and catch prey while avoiding predators—all the while breathing air with 50 percent oxygen. Movement and activity improves blood and lymphatic circulation and the ability of the lungs to use oxygen.

Nowadays, as we're breathing 21 percent oxygen, we've become a generation of couch potatoes. Maybe now that you understand the importance of oxygen, you'll have a different outlook on walking, running, and playing with your pets. When you engage in physical activity, you're increasing respiration and blowing out carbon dioxide, which creates a more oxygenated and alkaline body—so you're pursuing not only better physical fitness but also a healthier, more oxygenated body.

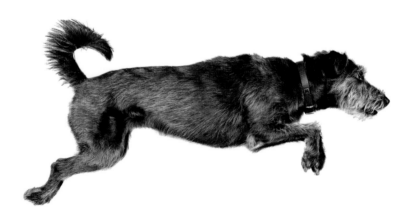

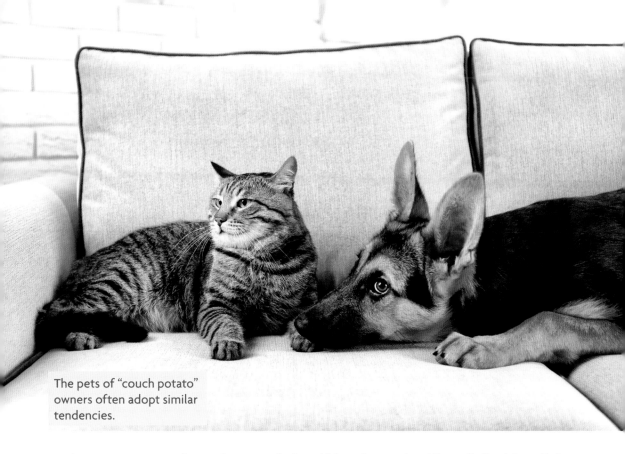

The pets of "couch potato" owners often adopt similar tendencies.

When you measure a substance's pH, you find out if the substance is *acidic* or *alkaline* (also called *basic*). In high school science, you may have learned about pH using little strips of paper called *litmus paper*. These paper strips would turn various shades of red or blue after being soaked in liquid, thus indicating the pH of that liquid. You would have found that vinegar and lemon juice are acidic, and therefore taste sour, while baking soda is alkaline, and therefore tastes bitter.

So what does pH mean and why is it crucially important to health? The abbreviation *pH* stands for "potential hydrogen." The pH of any solution is the measure of its hydrogen-ion concentration. The higher the pH, the more *alkalkine* and the more *oxygen-rich* the fluid is. Let's say that again for emphasis: *oxygen-rich*.

Being oxygen-rich is the key to the health of cells and organs. Healthy functioning of the liver, pancreas, gallbladder, heart, kidneys, hormones, and all other organs and systems depends on alkaline conditions. The more alkaline the environment, the better everything in the body performs.

Cells are surrounded by an interstitial fluid, secreted by the cells themselves, that bathes and envelops them. An alkaline interstitial fluid allows organs, such as the kidneys and liver, to function far more efficiently.

The food your pet eats will determine the pH of his or her body. However, a food's pH, measured when it is sitting in a bowl on the counter, is not going to reflect the effect that the food will have

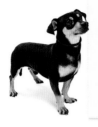

Did You Know?

When acid rain "kills" a lake, the fish literally suffocate to death because the acid in the lake binds up all of the available oxygen. It's not that the oxygen has gone anywhere; it's just no longer available.

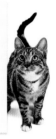

on the pH your dog's body. In fact, a food's original pH can have the opposite effect on the body. A food's pH effect on the body is determined *after it is digested*.

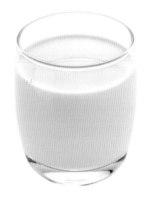

As one example, a lemon is acidic outside of the body but will, when eaten and digested, make the body's fluid more alkaline. Milk, an alkaline outside the body, will have the effect of making the body itself more acidic. Apple cider vinegar is, of course, acidic, but it will create an alkaline effect within the body. Fermented foods will also alkalinize cells and organs.

Meat, poultry, and similar protein sources have the effect of making the body more acidic. There's an interesting explanation of why this happens. When these proteins are digested, molecules of both sulfur and phosphorus are formed, making the intestinal tract acidic. Meat also contains nitrogen, which, when digested, transforms into ammonia. Ammonia is toxic to cells, so the body needs to neutralize all of it first and then excrete it.

The body does have a way to neutralize and manage excess acids and toxins: it uses its stores of bicarbonate. These bicarbonate stores are pulled into the gut to neutralize the acidic environment that's been created by the ammonia and other compounds in the intestinal tract. When these stores are released and lost into the bowels, the intracellular fluids—having lost their stores of bicarbonate—become acidic.

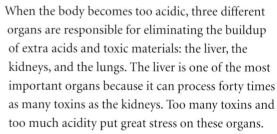

When the body becomes too acidic, three different organs are responsible for eliminating the buildup of extra acids and toxic materials: the liver, the kidneys, and the lungs. The liver is one of the most important organs because it can process forty times as many toxins as the kidneys. Too many toxins and too much acidity put great stress on these organs.

A Recipe for Cancer

- Acidic environment
- Carcinogens in meat and poultry
- Growth hormones in meat and poultry
- Vaccines

When the body is acidic, it cannot perform the tasks of maintenance, cleaning, and generating cellular ATP (adenosine triphosphate) adequately. Without ATP—the cells' source of energy—their batteries run low and carcinogens build up.

Our pets should eat foods that help alkalinize and oxygenate the cells and organs in their bodies. They should also be encouraged to exercise every day as part of this effort. Simple, everyday activities, often taken for granted, can have an important impact on the health of our pets.

Liver Detox: A "Spring Cleaning" for Dogs and Cats

Unfortunately, in today's world, our pets carry a heavy "toxic load" and their liver and kidneys are tasked with the job of clearing it all out as best they can. Chronic health problems can often result from a toxic load. More so than us humans, dogs and cats need to be detoxed. And that's particularly important in the springtime. Why?

Interestingly, in the spring, the pineal gland is stimulated by the increase in available natural light. As a result, the pineal gland stimulates the body to naturally detox. That's why horses eat strange and seemingly unpalatable greenery in the springtime—stuff they would never eat at the end of the summer.

Rather than being troubled about all of those dandelions on your lawn, you can use them to detoxify your pet's liver (see pages 78-79). Both the root and the leaves can be used for medicinal

Cats Gone Green

Let's face it: Cats and dogs are different, and that's why you need some tips on how to get greens–which will have an alkalinizing effect–into your cat. One is by way of kitty greens. You can find kits online that have everything you need to grow sequential pots of greens for your cat to munch. Once you see how it's done, you can grow these green shoots by getting some grains at the health-food store and seeding them into a plant pot. Cats also will often tolerate some chlorophyll or chlorella powder or liquid in their food, but usually you have to begin with small amounts.

Foods That Promote an Alkaline pH

Alfalfa	Broccoli	Dulce	Mustard greens
Apple cider vinegar	Cabbage	Garlic	Pears
	Cauliflower	Ginger	Pumpkin
Apples	Chard greens	Green beans	Spirulina
Bananas	Chlorella	Kale	Sweet potatoes
Barley greens	Cinnamon	Molasses, blackstrap	Watermelon
Beet greens	Collard greens		

purposes. The leaves work as a digestive and liver tonic; dandelion tonics have been used and are still used to clean and tone the liver and remove toxins from the bloodstream. The roots are used as a cleansing tonic for gallstones, jaundice, and constipation. Dandelion leaves are also specific medicine for the kidneys because they flush and tone these organs. Additionally, dandelions have been used successfully for dandruff, toothaches, sores, fevers, and rotting gums.

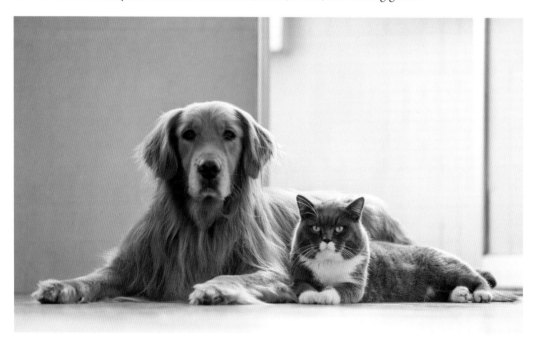

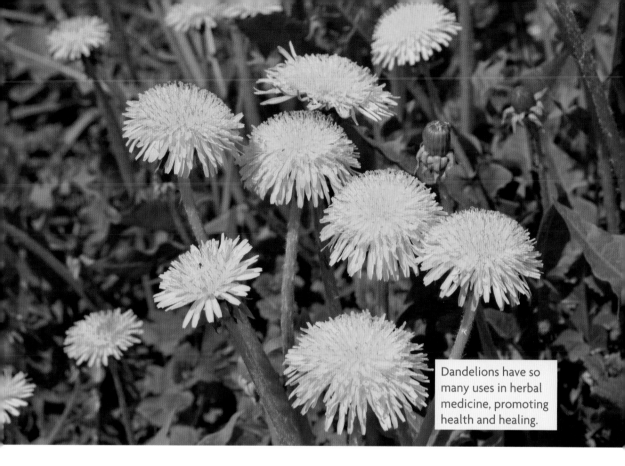

Dandelions have so many uses in herbal medicine, promoting health and healing.

Dandelions can taste bitter, so add them sparingly to your pet's diet at first, using the youngest shoots of plants that have not been sprayed with any type of chemicals. The best way to introduce them is to chop up a few young leaves and sauté them in butter. Then beat up a few eggs and make dandelion scrambled eggs for your dog (cats typically do not like dandelion greens).

You can also make a healing tea for your dog by placing two to three tablespoons of the leaves into one cup of water and bringing it to a boil. Simmer gently for fifteen minutes and then let cool. You can also make an infusion or tea by pouring hot water over the leaves and allowing the mixture to steep for five to thirty minutes. Give one tablespoon of the liquid three times a day to a medium-sized dog.

1. Spring Cleanse for Dogs

The easiest way to do a spring cleanse is to get capsules of dried whole dandelion from a reputable source. Give the capsules wrapped in something tasty before a meal twice a day.

Large dogs can take the recommended human dose; medium-sized dogs can take half of the human dose, and small dogs can take one-quarter of the human dose. Start when the weather begins to get warmer in February, March, or April and give the dandelion for two weeks up to one month.

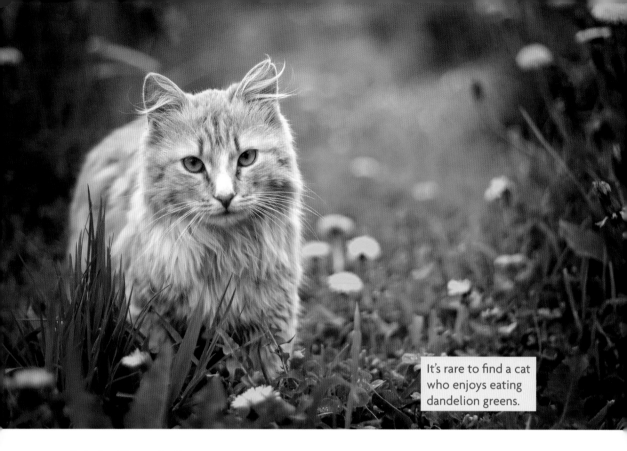

It's rare to find a cat who enjoys eating dandelion greens.

2. Spring Cleanse for Cats

If you have a cat who likes dandelion leaves, please call me—I want to frame her picture! The same homeopathic remedies that we have used for dogs can be given to cats for a month in the spring, and that's pretty easy. The section on instructions for administering homeopathic remedies (page 210) will show you how to do this.

If you already give your cat kitty greens, chlorophyll, or chlorella all year 'round, you're in pretty good shape. Just add the homeopathic remedies to the mix. If you don't regularly offer greens, I suggest adding them for at least a month.

3. Homeopathic Remedies for Springtime Liver Cleanse

Give a combination of Ptelea 6x, Taraxacum 6x, and Carduus marianus 6x orally, twice a day for one month. These three homeopathic remedies are specific for cleansing the liver. For instructions on how to give homeopathic remedies go to page 210.

The Important Intestine

Your pet's gut is essential to his or her overall health and immune-system function. The small intestine is actually like a garden that nurtures and grows good bacteria and prevents the growth of pathogenic bacteria.

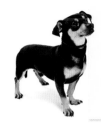

Did You Know?

Areas of the small intestine are called Peyer's patches, and they contain many small masses of lymphatic tissue, similar to lymph nodes.

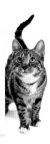

The digestive tract is an important component of our pets' immune systems. In fact, 80 percent of our dogs' and cats' immune systems sit right in their Peyer's patches.

This makes it easier to understand how immunity is related to intestinal health. The immune system of the intestinal tract is called GALT: gut-associated lymphoid tissue. Throughout the intestinal tract, there are macrophages and lymphocytes positioned immediately under the intestinal lining cells as well as deeper in the intestinal tissue along with Peyer's patches.

The gut contains thousands of strains of bacteria. After just a single course of antibiotics, the strong bacteria come back, but the less hardy varieties will never return. Researchers are now learning that these more minor bacteria actually hold important functions in T-cell activation.

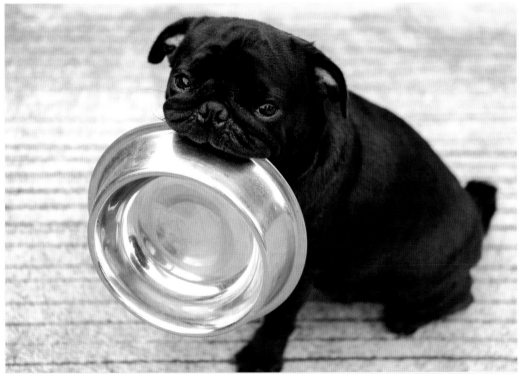

Intestinal health plays a large role in your pet's overall health.

The gut flora is the foundation of the immune system, but modern lifestyles have totally changed the composition of this flora in both humans and their pets. A study of primitive people in Brazil, who have never taken antibiotics and do not consume sugar, white flour, or processed foods, shows that they have a very different composition of friendly flora in their guts.

There exists within the gut a number of components that are integral to the health of the gut and, thus, the immune system.

Glucans: Gut Communication

The body doesn't produce glucans naturally. The only way to get the compound is from outside sources, such as baker's yeast, mushrooms, and cereal grains like barley, oats, and rye. Decades of research shows that glucans have a significant role in stimulating defense reactions against infections and cancer. Special cells in the gut facilitate the transport of glucans across the intestinal wall into the Peyer's patches, where they interact with macrophages to activate immune function.

Macrophage interaction enhances the production, size, and function of NK (natural killer) cells, T-cells, and B-cells. These cells, as a matter of course, are necessary to wage war against bacteria, microbes, viruses, and fungi. Glucans are polysaccharides, and there are hundreds of different combinations of polysaccharide compounds. Some of these polysaccharides are effective in protecting against cancer while all of them improve the immune function of the gut.

Transfer Factors: Gut Education

Transfer factors are tiny molecules that intelligently regulate immune-system activities. Transfer factors understand the dialogue of all cells. These molecules transfer immune memory and knowledge from one cell to another. They educate the immunoglobulin A, the helper T-cells, and the NK cells in the Peyer's patches of the gut. As an oral dietary supplement, they're derived from colostrum or chicken egg yolk.

Probiotics: The Facilitators

Over half of the stool is made up of beneficial gut bacteria, which play a huge part in the body's health. In fact, the intestine is just an extension of the skin, and each part of the digestive tract has a purpose. The gut flora is the foundation of the immune system. One might even call the gut flora the "canary in the coal mine."

There are thousands of strains of bacteria in the gut, so maintaining gut flora with probiotics in food and supplements becomes a complicated job. Combining effective probiotics with attention to the purposes of each strain can seem nearly impossible. One guru of human probiotic therapy said that the deeper you get into probiotics, the more confused you get. I can't disagree.

There are multiple considerations at work.

- The strains present in probiotic formulations vary widely.
- Some probiotics cannot last on store shelves for more than six months.
- Many strains of bacteria, such as lactose, live only eight days after being seeded in the gut, while some strains, such as the bifidos, are stronger bacteria that return after antibiotic treatment.
- Do probiotics (if they are still alive when you purchase and ingest them) actually make it to the gut?

Research indicates that anywhere from 80 to 99 percent of traditional, unprotected, live probiotic cells will be killed off by stomach acid before reaching the intestine. In order for the good bacteria to provide their beneficial effects, they must be able to survive in numbers high enough to allow them to do their jobs.

A process in which the probiotic is coated in a substance to protect it from acid has been tested and proven to shield it from the damaging effects of stomach acid and bile. Probonix is one brand of probiotics prepared this way, and they make palatable formulas for both dogs and cats.

Prebiotics are as important as, if not more important than, probiotics because they provide the nutrition that the good bacteria need to survive and thrive. Simple green vegetables and herbs, like artichoke, asparagus, and dandelion greens, are all excellent prebiotics. Pectin is also a prebiotic—remember, "an apple a day keeps the doctor away."

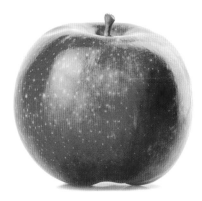

Probiotic Considerations

In order for the good bacteria to provide their beneficial effects, they must be able to survive in numbers high enough to allow them to do their jobs. The way that most traditional probiotic products are processed and packaged does not promote high survival rates. These supplements often claim billions of active cells per dose on their labels, but they do not promise whether these probiotic cells will stay alive and healthy once they enter the intestines. Additionally, while they are active right after processing, how do we know if they are still active or even alive when you take it off the store shelf?

A process in which the probiotics are coated to protect them from acid has been tested and proven to work against the damaging effects of stomach acid and bile, delivering live probiotic cultures.

Probiotic bacteria have a four-phase life cycle:

1. Lag phase: In the beginning, the bacteria are dormant, not replicating. They are not consuming food and are simply adapting to their environment.

2. Growth phase: The bacteria are replicating exponentially and using up nutrients in their environment. They are also generating much waste, such as acids, as a by-product of their replication process.

3. Static phase: The growth has plateaued because much of the available nutrients have been used up.

4. Death phase: Self-explanatory.

Probiotics are sold in all four phases. Those in the lag phase typically do not require refrigeration because they are dormant, not growing or consuming nutrients. However, live bacteria in the growth phase typically require refrigeration because they are packaged with a food source (e.g., simple sugars) and have already started growing. The purpose of refrigeration is to slow down their metabolism so they do not consume all of their food while sitting in the stores, waiting to be purchased and ingested. Now imagine what happens when the bacteria run out of food: they plateau and reach a static phase, followed by death, all before you even take the supplement.

Probiotics that *do not* require refrigeration have a longer shelf life and may have a better chance of surviving once ingested. This makes sense because the bacteria are only in the first phase, the lag phase. So, to spend your money wisely, it just makes sense to go with the supplements that will remain potent longer, right? This means they are more likely to do the job you want them to do.

Unrefrigerated probiotic supplements that contain bacteria in the lag phase do not need to be manufactured or coated with a food source because they are not actively dividing. Being in the lag phase, and being able to adapt to an acidic environment, helps the bacterial cultures better survive through the stomach acid, as they have already adapted to this type of acidic conditions.

In summary, probiotics are confusing—even to the experts. Every single year, more and more is learned about the, literally, thousands of strains that live in our gut. Probiotic combinations vary in the strains they carry and in their mode of preparation and viability.

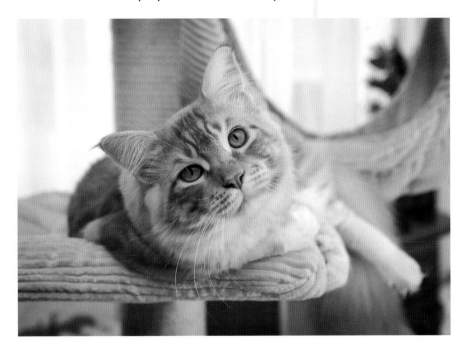

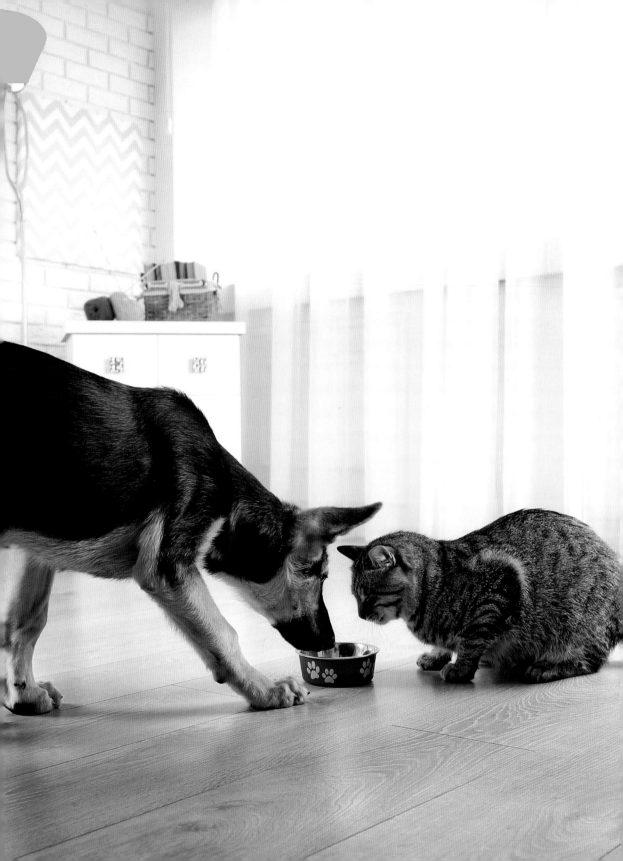

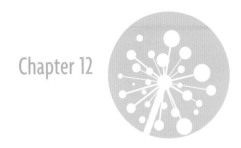

Chapter 12

Food:
Decoding the Mystery

*F*ood allergies and sensitivities can cause itching, GI problems, or both. Adding in environmental factors, such as mold, dust, and pollen adds insult to injury. It all adds up. However, because components in the food are just about always the major factor, changing the diet, when done with foresight and careful planning, can often help your pet.

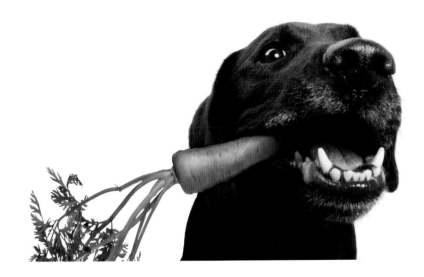

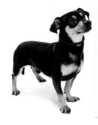

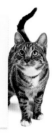

The information in this section will help resolve the confusion and frustration you've likely felt in attempting to find the food(s) that work for your pet. You also may feel a sense of helplessness. That's why I want you to know that there are real, curative solutions to both skin and GI problems. The Allergy Elimination 4 Pets technique, which you'll learn about later, can be a real lifesaver, and there are other options as well. We're going to discuss dietary fixes here, but no matter which methods and modalities you choose to apply, you'll need to understand everything in this section so you can prevent the problem from reoccurring once it's fixed.

If you recall our earlier discussion on phenolics, you understand that they are present in foods and in the environment and are likely culprits for both skin and gastrointestinal reactions. The facts that one phenolic can be present in many different foods and that one food can contain many phenolics make finding the right foods very tricky, if not impossible. For example, beef has ten different phenolics, while chicken has five.

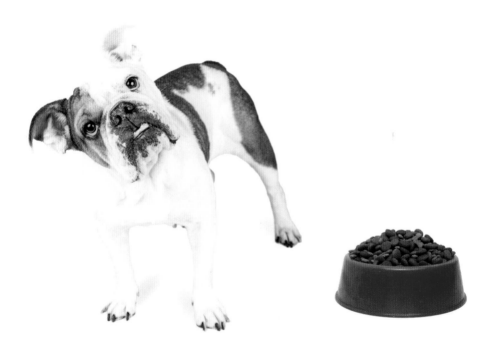

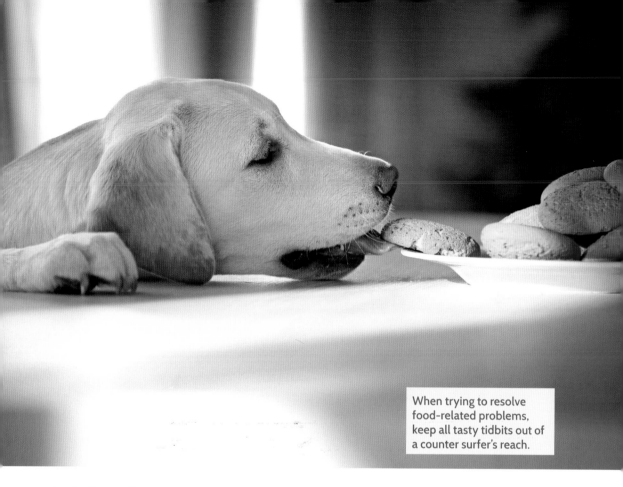

When trying to resolve food-related problems, keep all tasty tidbits out of a counter surfer's reach.

To further confuse matters, the delayed response produced by a sensitivity or intolerance works to confound us as we look to make dietary changes. Remember, food sensitivities and intolerances create a different type of response than allergies. The response is caused by the antibodies immunoglobulin A (IgA) and immunoglobulin M (IgM), which live in the *gut mucosa*, and the resulting inflammation and irritation take more than a week to develop. This makes it even more difficult to know if a new food that you're trying is really working. In addition, you have to wait a few weeks for all of the old food to leave the pet's intestinal crypts. Keeping a calendar of responses and having patience definitely help when trying to analyze the effects of changes to your pets' diet.

Commercial pet foods have many different ingredients. With processed pet foods, you need to take into account the colorings, preservatives, palatability enhancers, and other additives that most pet foods contain. Any or all of the compounds in these ingredients can cause a reaction, which means that a new diet with a different protein source may still contain problematic compounds.

Further, your pet can have reactions to ingredients in the supplements you're giving him or her in the hopes of resolving the allergy or intolerance. For example, I've found that giving fish oil for the omega-3 fatty acids rarely resolves the problem. Rather, the pet simply becomes reactive, sensitive, intolerant, or allergic to fish.

What's *Really* in Our Wheat?

Sometimes, what you think is a food allergy or intolerance is actually a reaction to a toxin. One example is wheat. Many people think that their pets are gluten-intolerant or allergic to wheat, but very few dogs and cats are actually gluten-intolerant. We know that wheat contains gallic acid–a major culprit as far as allergies go–but so do a lot of other foods that we commonly feed our dogs and cats. So why has wheat suddenly become the "bad guy?"

Something has been going on with wheat that goes far beyond the often-mentioned organic, hybridization, and gluten factors. And it clears up a mystery I've long been trying to solve.

Dogs have been eating the same thing as humans have for well over 10,000 years. At the same time, dogs have evolved alongside humans, becoming domesticated and living lives that are quite different from those of their wild wolf cousins. A lot has changed in the canine genetic makeup over that time period. As our dogs have coevolved with us, they've adapted to be able to digest the same diet as ours.

Novel adaptations in dogs' genes allowed the ancestors of our modern dogs to digest and assimilate starches. In fact, there's some pretty impressive genetic research that's been done in Sweden on this very subject.

Eric Axelsson, an evolutionary geneticist at Uppsala University in Sweden, compared the DNA from dogs and wolves. Unlike wolves, dogs had developed genes for digesting starch. Dogs have up to thirty copies of the gene that makes amylase, a protein that starts the breakdown of starch in the intestine, while wolves have only two copies. In addition, the multiple genes for amylase are twenty-eight times more active in dogs, showing that our canine friends are much better at digesting starches than wolves.

There's also another gene that codes for an additional enzyme–maltase–that is important in the digestion of starch. It was found that dogs produce a longer version of the maltase digestive enzyme than wolves. In fact, it's the same type of elongated version seen in herbivores, such as cows and rabbits, making it even more efficient in its ability to digest starch.

The bottom line is that dogs can eat and digest starches, they've developed enzymes, and they've adapted to a diet that's quite similar to a balanced human diet. So why are wheat and other grains now spurned in pet foods? Why did wheat suddenly become the "enemy" ingredient?

Let's start with the difficulty that farmers face when they harvest wheat. The kernels of wheat need to be as ripe as possible, and each stalk has many kernels. However, a wheat field ripens unevenly. To fix this problem, many wheat farmers in the United States spray their fields generously with herbicides containing the active ingredient glyphosate about a week before harvest. This allows the kernels to dry out evenly, leaving the farmers with easier harvests and higher yields. The use of glyphosate for this purpose steadily increased over the years until it became a very common protocol.

Farmers call the use of glyphosate with wheat *dessication*. Other crops, such as peas or lentils, would not be acceptable in the marketplace if sprayed with glyphosate pre-harvest. Certain European countries have banned glyphosate, and other places have designated glyphosate as a cancer-causing chemical, but we have to consider that wheat grown in the United States is sent all over the world. The Food Standards Agency in the United Kingdom reports that glyphosate residues regularly show up in bread samples. Today, 99 percent of durum wheat—the most common type of wheat—is treated with herbicides. Interestingly, many people who consider themselves gluten-intolerant find that when they eat bread made from wheat from countries that ban glyphosate, such as Italy and France, they have no ill effects from the wheat they consume.

Of course, herbicide manufacturers tout their products as being safe. But two researchers, Dr. Stephanie Seneff and Anthony Samsel of Massachusetts Institute of Technology, strongly argue in research published in the journal *Entropy* in April 2013 that glyphosate is not safe and that the consumption of this herbicide is greatly contributing to increases in many diseases. Most of the non-organic wheat supply is now contaminated with glyphosate.

Glyphosate is known to inhibit cytochrome P450 enzymes. Cytochrome P450 enzymes are involved in eliminating environmental toxins, activating vitamin D3, catabolizing vitamin A, and maintaining bile acid production and sulfate supplies to the gut. The good, beneficial intestinal bacteria are also rendered impotent by glyphosate. A large percentage of processed foods are made from wheat, and this helps explain the explosion of gastrointestinal problems.

Did You Know?

Today, many dogs and cats are vitamin D3 deficient. The good gut bacteria activate vitamin D3.

To quote the April 2013 article in *Entropy*: "CYP enzymes play crucial roles in biology, one of which is to detoxify xenobiotics. Thus, glyphosate enhances the damaging effects of other food-borne chemical residues and environmental toxins. Negative impact on the body is insidious and manifests slowly over time as inflammation damages cellular systems throughout the body. Here, we show how interference with CYP enzymes acts synergistically with disruption of the biosynthesis of aromatic amino acids by gut bacteria, as well as impairment in serum sulfate transport. Consequences are most of the diseases and conditions associated with a Western diet, which include gastrointestinal disorders, obesity, diabetes, heart disease, depression, autism, infertility, cancer, and Alzheimer's disease. We explain the documented effects of glyphosate and its ability to induce disease, and we show that glyphosate is the 'textbook example' of exogenous semiotic entropy: the disruption of homeostasis by environmental toxins."

You're getting it straight from the horse's mouth. Glyphosate significantly disrupts the functioning of the beneficial bacteria in the gut and contributes to the permeability of the intestinal wall. And the gut accounts for close to three-quarters of the body's immune function.

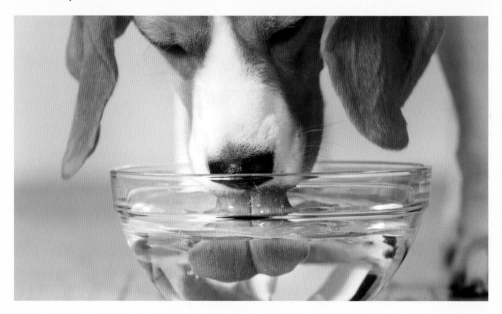

Did You Know?

Glyphosate is also used on barley, sugar cane, rice, sweet potato, sugar beets, and soy crops.

It's important to understand that you cannot wash glyphosate off foods because it is incorporated into each cell of the plant. The only way to truly handle this is to choose as many organic foods as possible for you and your pets. Organic standards do not permit the use of glyphosate. This consideration is equally as important, if not more important, when it comes to meat and other animal products; as factory-farmed animals are typically raised on a genetically modified (GMO) diet, so glyphosate bioaccumulates in their tissues. Do not confuse "organic" with "all-natural." The latter is not regulated and often contains GMO ingredients.

Once upon a time, all people and animals ate organic food, with most of it ripening on the vine. The phytonutrients, vitamins, and minerals in the plants worked to promote health and even cure disease. In today's world, we're all exposed to more than our fair share of carcinogens and other toxins. We need the ingredients in conscientiously grown food to eliminate these toxins and repair the damage they have done. It's more important than ever that we buy organic and fight for our rights to healthy food.

The long and short of it is that I recommend staying far away from wheat—and any other foods—that are sprayed with glyphosate before being harvested.

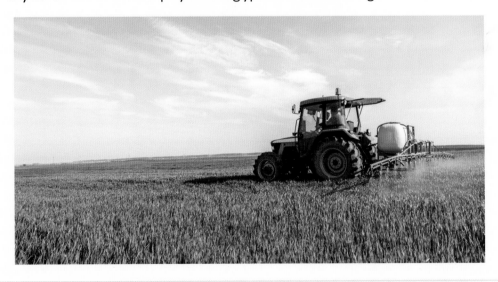

The Meat of the Matter

I'd like to pose a question: Could substances added to our meat in the United States be increasing the rate of cancer in our pets?

What you may not realize is that most mass-produced meat in the United States is injected with hormones and antibiotics. That's why imports of US meats are banned by the European Union, Russia, Australia, Canada, China, Taiwan, and Japan.

In 1999, a European Union scientific committee revealed that it had evidence to show that a growth hormone used in US cattle production is a "complete carcinogen." The committee warned that other hormones in US meats could also cause a variety of health problems. Then, a second report by the committee alleged "abusive" use and inadequate control of six growth hormones in the United States.

The FDA-approved hormones used to fatten up livestock (without having to feed them additional food) include recombinant bovine growth hormone [rbGH], estrogen, testosterone, and progesterone. It's estimated that the nontherapeutic use of antibiotics (to fatten animals up, not to treat or prevent disease) in livestock production accounts for nearly 80 percent of all antibiotics used in the United States. Importantly, antibiotics fed to livestock is the main reason we are and have been seeing so many deadly antibiotic-resistant bacteria.

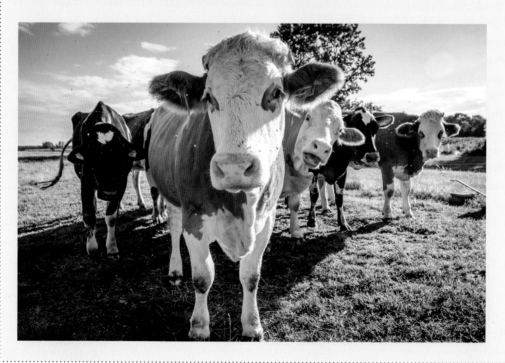

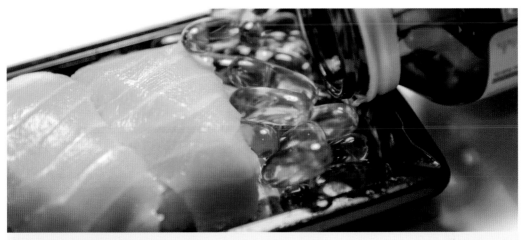

Pets may develop sensitivities to fish or fish-oil supplements.

There are many hypoallergenic diets available for our pets, and more and more commercial pet-food companies are developing novel food combinations. If you haven't been feeding your dog or cat a fish-based food or supplementing with fish oils, fish is often a good protein to start with. Remember though, that many cat foods are flavored with fish. That means that even if the food says "chicken" or "beef" on the label, reading the ingredients will reveal that fish has been added to spruce up the flavor. I also often recommend a rabbit-based food for both cats and dogs.

There are many tests that attempt to discern what your dog or cat may be allergic to. The most common is serum allergy testing. These tests can be 80 percent accurate for environmental allergies, but, unfortunately, they are not very accurate for foods. Knowing that foods are the Achilles heel of allergic symptoms, we can understand how these tests leave much to be desired.

To perform serum allergy testing, once your pet's potential allergens are identified, a special serum containing these allergens is formulated for your pet. But if you check out the relatively small sampling of trees, grasses, weeds, molds, and foods that are tested for, you can see why the time and money spent on this type of testing and desensitization program doesn't often get you too far. Many of my patients who come to me with itchy skin or digestive problems have already gone this route with no results.

Dr. Jean Dodds has developed a test to identify food sensitivities in both dogs and cats called NutriScan® (*www.nutriscan.org*). It tests the most common foods eaten by dogs and cats by measuring the reaction of the IgA and IgM in the pet's saliva to pure extracts of these foods. NutriScan actually tests for food allergens and the resultant intolerances. In fact, these antibodies to foods appear in the saliva several months before the GI-tract diagnosis of IBD.

With NutriScan, all you have to do is get the kit and mail in your pet's saliva sample. Because food sensitivities change over time, you should repeat the test once or twice per year. The treatment is to change your pet's diet based on the test results, which tell you which foods to avoid and which foods are fine to feed to your pet.

Did You Know?

Studies have irrefutably shown that antibiotics cause weight gain. If you take a course of antibiotics and are surprised to find that you've put on a few pounds, that could be the very reason.

We can also see that these hormones in the foods we eat are certainly affecting our children. A study published in the September 2010 issue of the medical journal *Pediatrics* reveals a surprisingly big increase in the numbers of girls beginning puberty between the ages of seven and eight.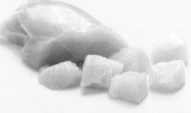

But what about our dogs and cats? What about all of the cancer we're seeing? One answer is found in a study published in 1999 in the *Journal of Clinical Oncology*, stating that eating foods with natural or synthetic insulin-like growth factor-1 (IGF-1) may be linked to an increase in certain cancers, including prostate, breast, and colon cancers.

Andrew Weil, MD, has stated that more than two-thirds of the cattle raised in the U.S. are given hormones, usually testosterone and estrogen, to boost growth. According to a fact sheet published by Cornell University in June 2000, there are six FDA-approved steroid hormones commonly used in meat and dairy production in the United States: estradiol, progesterone, testosterone, zeranol, trenbolone acetate, and melengestrol. The FDA also allows the use of rbGH to promote more milk production in dairy cows.

Research certainly shows that growth hormones increase cancer. In addition to the previously mentioned cancers, growth hormones increase the risk of Hodgkin's lymphoma, a B-cell lymphoma. Lymphoma, or lymphosarcoma, is a cancer of the lymph nodes or GI tract that occurs in dogs and cats, and, in my clinical experience, is becoming all too common in our pets. Our furry best friends tend to eat a lot more meat and poultry than we do.

All too often, I see owners of dogs and cats with food sensitivities and allergies jump to an all-meat diet. For some, it works well, because fresh food is better than processed kibble any day. But for many, it doesn't help at all. Remember when we talked about phenolics and how one particularly troublesome phenolic, gallic acid, was in so many foods? If gallic acid was the culprit in your dog's or cat's problems, changing to a raw diet is like jumping from the frying pan into the fire. Additionally, if you do not add alkaline veggies and fruits to the diet, you're creating a very acidic environment.

Did You Know?

Itchy, allergic dogs suffer from intense itching and often redness of and papules on the skin, particularly on the belly, legs, face and ears. This is often coupled with inflammation of the nasal cavity and eyes, especially in response to seasonal changes.

In a small but promising study published by C.J Klinger et al in the *British Veterinary Record* (April 7, 2018), significant improvements were reported in dogs diagnosed with this condition and given a high oral dose of vitamin D3. Starting with 300 international units (IU) per 1 kg body weight and increasing to 1,400 IU over a four-week period, the high intake was maintained with veterinary monitoring. Vitamin D3 benefits have been reported for people with this skin condition and also asthma, hypertension, congestive heart failure, cancer, and dementia.

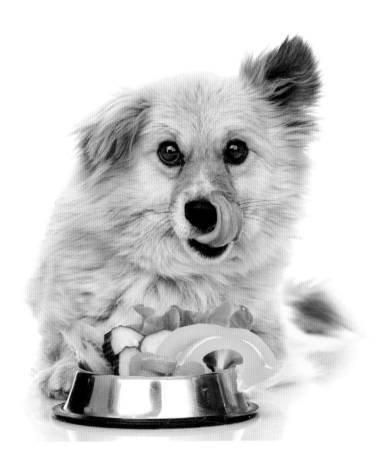

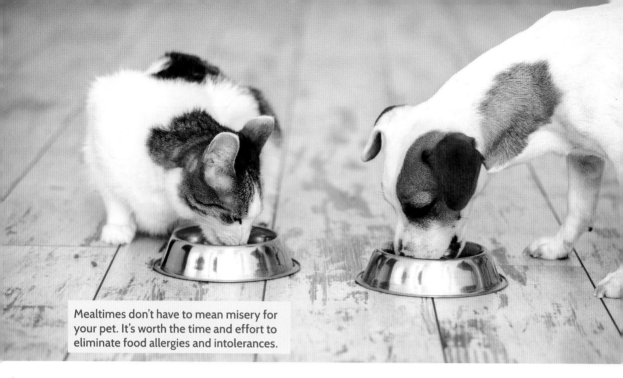

Mealtimes don't have to mean misery for your pet. It's worth the time and effort to eliminate food allergies and intolerances.

Later in the book, we're going to be talking about the Allergy Elimination 4 Pets technique. This is a holistic technique that finds your pet's allergies, sensitivities, and intolerances and then reprograms your pet's immune response so that he or she no longer has any reactions to anything. This program, which you do at home, normalizes your pet's reactions to both food and environmental culprits and then—*voilà*—you have a normal, healthy pet with no allergies. Stories like those at the beginning of the book are common, and now these pets lead full and normal lives with no dietary restrictions. For you, this means no more running from food to food, reading ingredients with a magnifying glass and cross-checking every snack you feed your dog or cat.

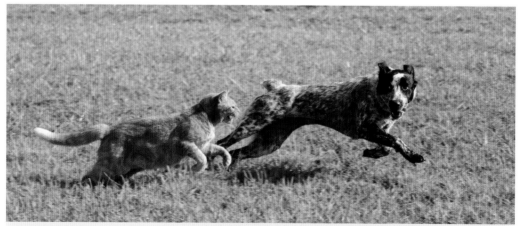

A proper diet with no sensitivities means energy and freedom from chronic symptoms for your pet.

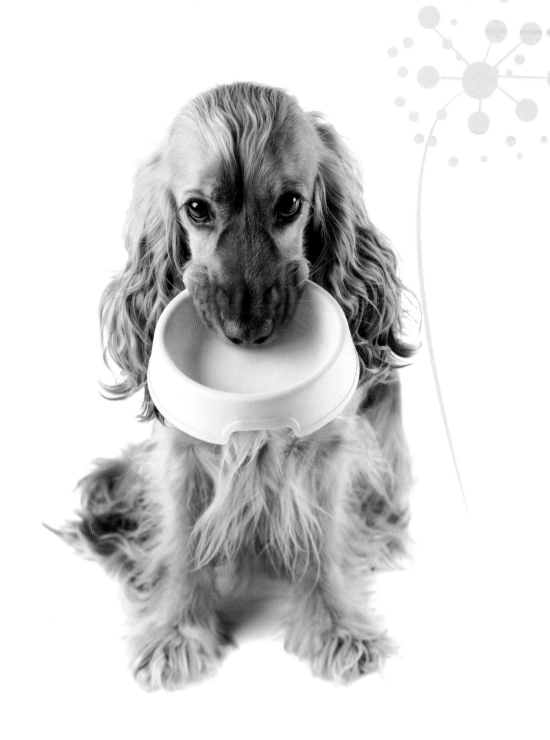

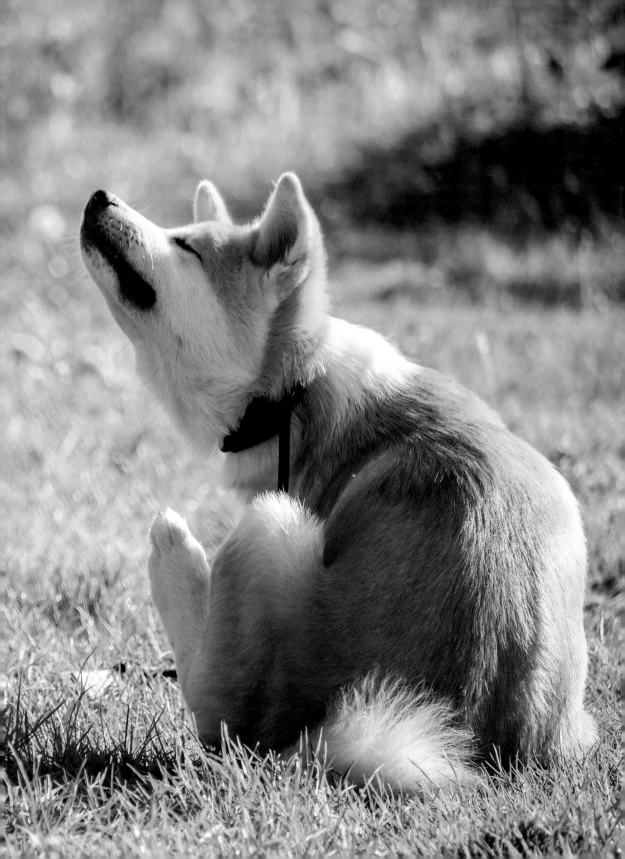

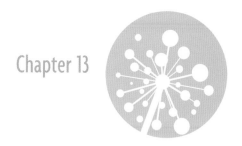

Chapter 13

Fixing the Itch:
The Natural Approach

When you were a child, your mother might have told you to stop scratching your mosquito bite because the scratching would only make it worse. It all comes down to the body's histamine response.

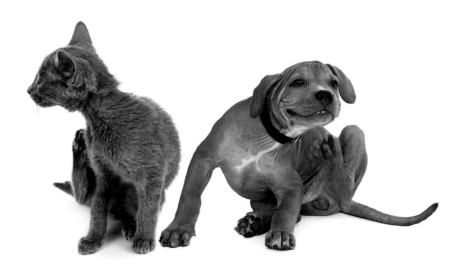

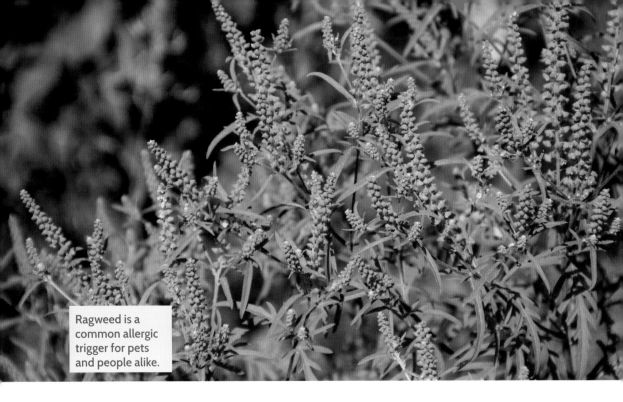

Ragweed is a common allergic trigger for pets and people alike.

Topical Tips to Stop the Itch

It's a vicious cycle: scratching irritates mast cells, which produce histamine during inflammatory and allergic reactions, and scratching compounds the problem by further intensifying the itch. If we compare humans with our dogs and cats, we'll find that our pets have ten times as many mast cells in their skin as we do. That means that they experience a lot more itching with any kind of allergic response.

Additionally, the histamine-producing mast cells are spread all over our pets' bodies. If we were set up just like our pets, ragweed season would have us scratching our inner thighs, butts, and chests while remarking to our coworkers how bad the ragweed was that day.

A good strategy is to apply a remedy that will stop the itch quickly and prevent the escalation of histamine in the tissues. The good news is that there are many readily available natural topical products that will do the job well. In fact, you may have many of these itch fixes already in your home. When you nip the itch in the bud, the problem is most likely to get resolved unless it's a systemic issue.

Calendula Officinalis

This herb is a favorite first aid treatment among herbalists, and for good reason. It has an almost magical effect in healing wounds. Calendula has a more powerful ability to hinder bacteria than many antibiotics, and it also has the important benefit of an anti-inflammatory effect while promoting the healthy growth of new cells. It also helps eliminate fungal infections.

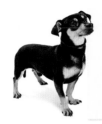
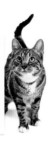

Did You Know?

Baking-soda paste is very helpful with dogs
who have itchy, irritated feet. Put the paste
between the toes and on the tops of the feet.

The Romans coined the name *calendula* to reflect the herb's blooming schedule because it would flower on the *calends*, or new moon, of every month. *Officinalis* refers to its official medicinal value. Calendula tincture diluted with water from 1:5 to 1:10 is effective and dependable for the treatment of itchy spots, and it can stop a hot spot in its tracks. You can buy tincture of calendula from a health food store or an herbal or homeopathic supply store. After diluting and mixing the tincture, apply it with a spray bottle or just pour some on the area and rub it in.

Alternatively, you can steep dried calendula petals to make your own tincture. Pour a cup of boiling water onto five tablespoons of calendula petals and steep for fifteen minutes. This tincture does not have to be diluted the way a purchased tincture does.

Baking Soda

Baking soda can work wonders! It has a soothing effect due to its anti-inflammatory properties. Plus, it acts as an acid neutralizer and creates a more basic pH that truly helps relieve itching. It's easy and very effective; plus, baking soda is safe, it does not stain, and it can be vacuumed up easily if it dries and flakes off.

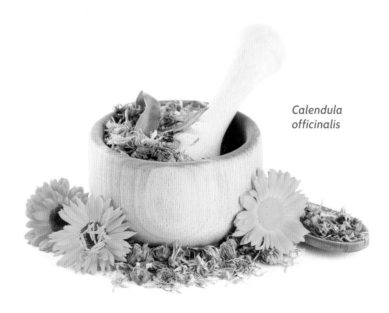

Calendula officinalis

Mix one tablespoon of baking soda with a little water to make a paste. Place the paste on your pet's areas itchy or reddened areas. Leave the paste on for a few hours and then wash it off. You can also make a baking soda spray by mixing two tablespoons of baking soda with eight ounces of water. Pour the mixture into a spray bottle and use when necessary. Shake before using.

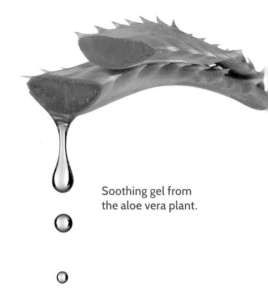

Soothing gel from the aloe vera plant.

Aloe Vera

There's a real difference between aloe vera gel you can buy in the store and that which comes from the live plant. The live plant has important enzymes that last for less than three days in the refrigerator. These special enzymes are incredibly powerful and work rapidly to heal itchy skin, but they are not present in bottled aloe vera gel.

Each aloe leaf contains a jellylike substance that rapidly regenerates damaged tissue; it also contains antibiotic and coagulating agents and can be used for wounds, fungal infections, and insect bites in addition to itchy areas. Gel from the aloe plant increases the rate of healing in the cellular matrix and decreases inflammation.

Obtain fresh aloe gel by splitting a leaf. Use the hard cuticle of the leaf to apply the green-tinged jelly inside the leaf to itchy areas. If you cut a leaf and use only part of it, store the rest of it in the refrigerator. Remember—after the leaf is cut, the ingredients will remain active for less than three days.

You can find aloe plants at nurseries and garden centers, and they are easy to maintain in your home. Place a terra-cotta pot with an aloe vera plant on your windowsill, and it will always be available to you.

Witch Hazel

Witch hazel, also known as winter-bloom or spotted alder, is a flowering shrub common in North America. The leaves, bark, and twigs of witch hazel are high in tannins, which are found in any natural astringent because of their ability to tighten, dry, and harden tissues. Witch hazel liquid, easily and inexpensively purchased at any drugstore, is actually a steam distillation of the bark, leaves, and twigs of the witch hazel shrub. When applied directly to the skin, witch hazel helps soothe itchy skin, reduce swelling, repair broken skin, and fight bacteria.

Some other wonderful things about witch hazel are that it's 100 percent natural, it smells fresh, and it doesn't stain furniture or carpets when you apply it to your pet. To use, simply soak a cloth or cotton ball in witch hazel and rub it on your pet's skin. It's also great for itchy paws. You can put some witch hazel in a plastic bowl, dip your dog's feet in it, and then pat dry.

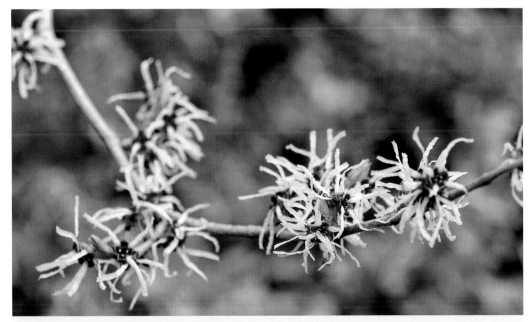
Witch hazel has astringent properties and can soothe irritated skin.

Grindelia Robusta and Grindelia Squarrosa

The administration of grindelia lies within the realm of homeopathy. You won't find this herb in the local drugstore or health food store. Grindelia tincture is made from the leaves and flowers of the Asteraceae (Compositae) family that grow on the United States' Pacific coast and inland in the mountains. The heads of the grindelia flowers get covered with a viscid balsamic secretion and thus have been called gumweed or rosin-weed.

Tincture of grindelia, after being diluted 1:10 with water, can be a very effective treatment for itching. You can order this tincture from a homeopathic supply store and dilute it before use.

You can either pour the mixture onto the itchy area, soak a cotton ball and apply it, or place the mixture in a spray bottle and spray the area. Apply as frequently as needed and watch the progress.

The homeopathic remedy Grindelia can also be used orally in a 6x or 6c potency. Give a few pellets or granules orally (you can tip them into your pet's cheek) and allow them to dissolve in his or her mouth. Homeopathic remedies should never be mixed into or given with food.

> ## Be Ready!
> If your pet tends to get itchy spots in the summer, I suggest having some of the remedies discussed in this chapter on hand and ready to go in your first aid kit so you can nip it in the bud.

Additional Remedies

While not every one of these natural remedies will work perfectly on every pet, there's a very good chance that most of them will work on most pets. If one solution isn't effective, don't hesitate to try another one.

Black tea or Japanese green tea: When prepared as a very strong brew, the resulting liquid can be applied to the inflamed area for three to ten minutes to soothe it. You can store the rest of the brew in the refrigerator and use it later.

Cabbage leaf: This old-time remedy works to remove heat and inflammation from an area. To apply, pound one cabbage leaf until the surface is broken so that the juice oozes out and then hold the leaf on the inflamed area. The leaf will begin to get warm as it soaks the inflammation out. Remove the leaf after several minutes.

Colloidal oatmeal: Found in pharmacies, colloidal oatmeal can be added to your pet's bath or used as a poultice.

Enzyme products: I personally love Zymox® LP3 enzymatic products for ear infections and itch relief. Only the mildest plant surfactants are used, and the enzymes have anti-inflammatory properties that calm the skin. The LP3 enzyme system delivers antimicrobial properties to infectious pus and debris. The bioactive enzymes are safe, effective, and nontoxic.

There is a Zymox spray with a little hydrocortisone, but one spritz often does the trick. For a pet who just won't stop bothering a specific area, it's worth it to use the spray with hydrocortisone.

Phenolic remedies: These include gallic acid and coumarin. Gallic acid, the most implicated phenolic for intolerances and insensitivities, is given at a rate of one drop, once a day, for two weeks; then two drops, twice a day, for two weeks; and then three drops, twice a day, for one month. Coumarin is also implicated in itching. Its dosage and frequency is the same as that of gallic acid.

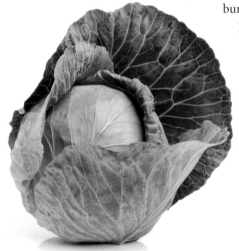

Preparation H cream: This cream stops itching and burning and often proves helpful with itchy skin. It is easy to find in drugstores and contains no harmful ingredients.

Zinc oxide ointment: This popular ingredient in diaper-rash ointment can work miracles in the right situations. It is great for treating areas where moisture collects and causes secondary infections, such as lip folds, the vaginal area, and folds at the base of the tail. I've had patients who saw their conventional veterinarians over and over again to no avail, but their pets' problems finally resolved after they began to apply zinc-oxide-based diaper-rash ointment.

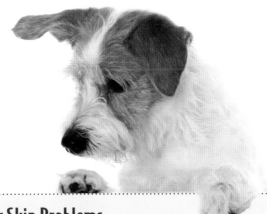

Homepathic Remedies for Skin Problems

Apis mellifica 6c–This is recommended for itching with hot, puffy sores or hives and sometimes facial swelling.

Arsenicum album 30x–Typically, this is used with a pet who is seeking heat because warmth relieves the itching. He or she has dry, scaly, itchy sores; is restless; and has intense itching even though the skin may appear normal.

Grindelia 30x–This is more of an acute remedy to slow the itching down while the other remedies begin to work. It can be given three times a day for several weeks with no problems.

Ledum 6x–This works to relieve itchiness from flea or tick bites.

Psorinum 200c–This is a deep-acting remedy for the skin, particularly skin that looks unhealthy and heals slowly. It's often a good remedy to make the body more receptive to other remedies, helping them work better. Unfortunately, it is not available in the United States, but it can be purchased overseas.

Rhus toxicodendron 6x–This remedy is made from poison ivy. It works for symptoms that resemble the rash and itchiness caused by the plant.

Silicea 30x–This works for recurrent skin infections with persistent but not intense itching, including infections that may begin after vaccination.

Sulfur 6c–This is a chief remedy to soothe itching in the pet that avoids heat and seeks cold. Bathing may aggravate the skin condition.

Thuja 6c–A key antivaccinosis remedy, this is indicated if skin problems began within weeks to months of vaccination. Also good with pets who tend to develop warts, have poor hair growth, and have skin that tends to become pigmented or turn black in areas.

Hot Tips for Hot Spots

The best approach with hot spots is to prevent recurrences by finding the underlying cause. Many things can cause hotspots: matted fur, a new shampoo, fleas and ticks, and allergies. Remember that our pets have many more of the specialized cells that cause inflammation in their skin than we do. We can compare their itchiness from a hot spot to what we experience when we have poison ivy.

The more the dog or cat bothers the area, the more it itches, and a vicious cycle begins. Further, hot spots can dramatically increase in size rapidly. What was the size of a quarter may double or triple in size in just a few hours. Redness, oozing, pain, and itchiness are the hallmark signs of hot spots, and hair loss is common. Sometimes hair can mat over the lesion, obscuring the size and degree of the problem.

Once a hot spot appears, you must treat it. The earlier you catch them, the faster they clear up. You may have to clip the hair from the surrounding area to administer treatment.

Topical Treatments

- Make a home remedy of baking soda and water mixed into a paste. Apply the paste to the irritated area and leave it on for a few hours before washing it off.
- Calendula tincture, a natural homeopathic remedy, can be diluted and sprayed onto the hot spot to provide relief and accelerate healing.

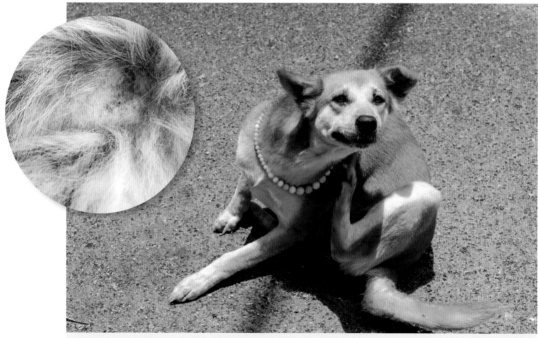

A hot spot causes itchiness and hair loss.

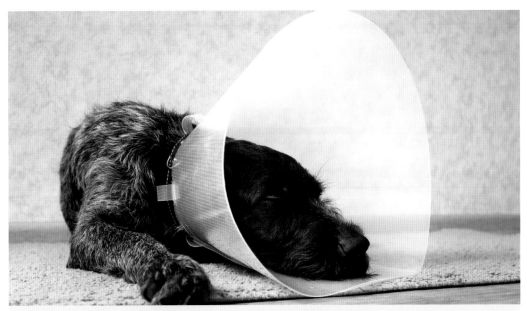

An Elizabethan collar, or "cone," prevents an animal from further damaging a hot spot or other wound.

- Fresh aloe vera directly from the leaf placed will soothe the irritated area immediately.
- Zymox spray with hydrocortisone is very dependable. A few spritzes one to three times over a half of a day and the problem is often solved.
- Colloidal silver spray works well if you catch the hot spot and start treatment early. You can combine colloidal silver spray with any of the other treatments listed.

Homeopathic Remedies for Hot Spots

Apis mellifica 6x—This remedy is recommended for areas that are swollen and very sensitive to touch. They can either look red or have a whitish hue. When pets need this remedy, they can show very little thirst. Give every few hours during the day for relief.

Belladonna 6c—Use when spots appear very quickly and are very intense. The spots are hot, red, and painful, and the pet can be more anxious than usual and more thirsty. Give every few hours until you notice relief.

Graphites 6c—Pets who need this remedy can have sticky honey-colored discharge from their hot spots. They can have a chilly disposition and tend to be overweight. Give this three times a day.

Hepar sulph 30c—With this remedy, the discharge may have a very noticeable odor. Give three times a day.

Mercurius sol 6c—Use with hotspots that tend to get a greenish discharge or a yellowish crust. Pustules that look like whitehead pimples may be present.

Rhus toxicodendron 6x—Use this remedy with hot spots that are more itchy than painful and may look like a poison ivy rash. The pet may be restless and may seem a bit stiff.

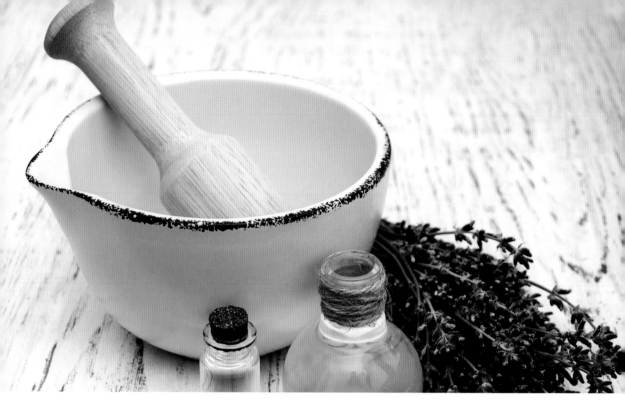

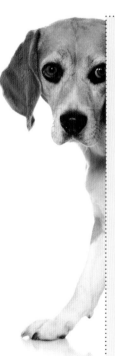

Lavender for Dogs

Lavender is known for its relaxing and soothing effect on the spirit, and it also works to reduce the buildup of excess oil on your dog's skin. You see, bacteria begin to grow in this excess oil, and it's actually the bacterial growth in the oil coat that's responsible for that musty odor that some dogs seem to have.

A lavender rinse after a bath or a few spritzes of lavender tea from a spray bottle works to decrease both the oil and the bacteria that grow in it, keeping odor at bay. As an added benefit, lavender is an anti-inflammatory and analgesic, so it decreases itchiness as well. It helps skin irritations and wounds because it promotes tissue regeneration and speeds up healing. Planted around the home, lavender works to repel flies and mosquitoes—not to mention that the delicate flowers are beautiful to look at and smell great!

Coat Refresher

½ cup lavender, chopped
4 cups water

Bring the water to a boil and add the lavender. Let the mixture steep for 30 minutes, strain, and then place enough for five days of use in a clean spray bottle. Refrigerate any remaining liquid. Spritz your dog's coat after a bath or in between baths to freshen up.

Allergy Rinse or Spray

2 tablespoons lavender leaves, chopped
2 tablespoons chamomile flowers and leaves, chopped
2 tablespoons calendula (marigold) petals, chopped
8 cups water

Bring the water to a boil. Place all of the dry ingredients in a pot and pour the boiling water over them. Let the pot sit on the stove over very low heat for 15 minutes. Remove from the heat and let the mixture cool for 45 minutes. Strain and pour the liquid into a clean jar or spray bottle and use it as a rinse or spray as needed.

Oil-Controlling Rinse or Spray

1 whole lemon, including skin and rind, sliced
4 tablespoons lavender leaves, coarsely chopped
6 cups water

Place all ingredients into an enamel or glass pot. Bring the mixture to a boil and simmer for 20 minutes. Remove the pot from heat and allow the entire mixture to sit overnight. Strain and store the liquid in a clean glass jar in the refrigerator. Use as an after-bath rinse or transfer to a spray bottle to spritz on the coat as needed.

Oil-Controlling Rinse or Spray

1 whole lemon, including skin and rind, sliced
4 tablespoons lavender leaves, coarsely chopped
6 cups water

Place all ingredients into an enamel or glass pot. Bring the mixture to a boil and simmer for 20 minutes. Remove the pot from heat and allow the entire mixture to sit overnight. Strain and store the liquid in a clean glass jar in the refrigerator. Use as an after-bath rinse or transfer to a spray bottle to spritz on the coat as needed.

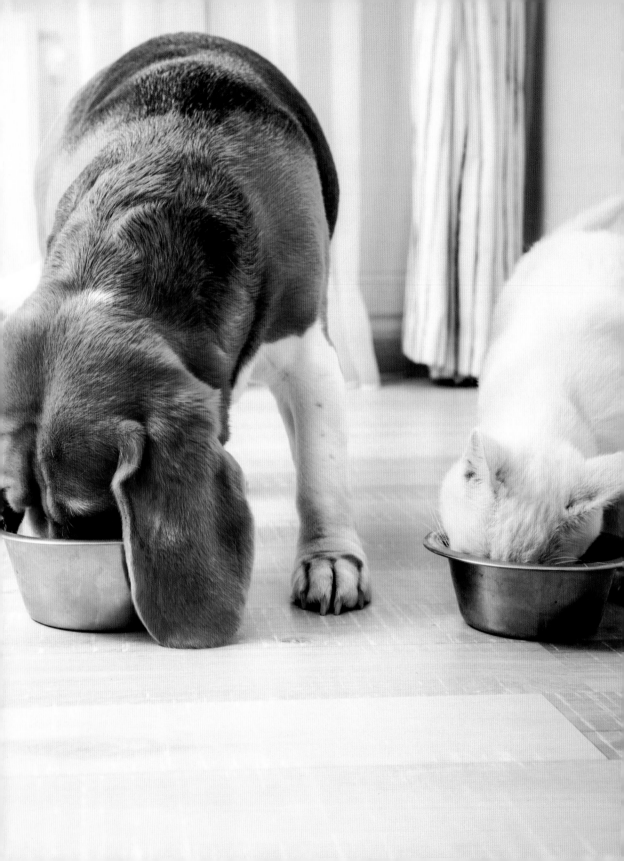

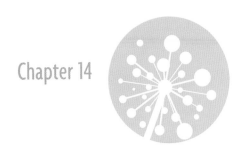

Chapter 14

Dealing with Gastrointestinal Problems: Natural Remedies for Diarrhea, Vomiting, and Constipation

$\mathcal{J}$ust as with skin problems, irritable bowel disease (IBD) and other chronic gastrointestinal problems are present in our dogs and cats in epidemic proportions, often caused by food sensitivities/intolerances. Perhaps you've simply decided that your dog or cat has a "sensitive" stomach. You may endlessly search for foods that will agree with his or her digestive system. Perhaps your pet has already been diagnosed with IBD. IBD can be viewed as a battleground in the gut, where the body's immune response struggles to defeat the invading armies of foreign substances.

Most commonly, pets with IBD have chronic diarrhea and vomiting, but after treating thousands of cases of IBD over the years, I've seen it all—from common symptoms to constipation and hiccupping. All of these pets were officially diagnosed by an intestinal biopsy. A biopsy in a pet with IBD will show a great increase in inflammatory cells in the digestive tract's lining.

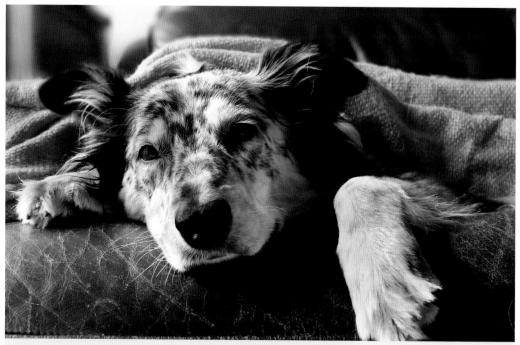

Gastrointestinal symptoms affect a pet's overall well-being and mood.

Basically, if your dog or cat has chronic diarrhea and/or chronic vomiting, which may or may not be accompanied by weight loss, there is a good chance he or she has IBD. That's because it's awfully likely that there are inflammatory responses in the lining of his or her digestive tract. You'll want to rule out intestinal parasites along with intestinal cancer as discussed in Chapter 10.

D3 and IBD

If your dog or cat has chronic diarrhea, you can be certain he or she is vitamin-D3 deficient. Let's find out just how important D3 is for the health of our furry friends.

Vitamin D3 has very important functions in the body. It affects mood and is an integral immune-system booster. One of the reasons people get fewer colds and bouts of flu in the summer is thought to be the increased levels—due to more sunlight—of this essential vitamin in their systems. The Department of International Health, Immunology, and Microbiology at the University of Copenhagen found that D3 activates the immune system's essential killer and helper cells, thus playing a major role in immune function. These cells can't even mobilize without adequate vitamin D. There is also a definite link between D3 deficiency and cancer.

Vitamin D3 deficiency in humans is now epidemic. People, unlike pets, get most of their D3 from UV exposure. When humans left the sunlight of the fields to work indoors and started using sunscreen when outside, their D3 levels suffered dramatically. It's now become routine to test human' vitamin D3 levels, supplementing this vitamin when necessary.

There are multiple factors that affect vitamin D3 status:

- While people get their vitamin D3 from UV radiation absorbed through the skin as well as from their diets, dogs and cats primarily get their form of active D3 from their diets.
- For pets over the age of five, vitamin D3 absorption drops by about 3 to 5 percent each year.
- The vitamin D3 levels of spayed female dogs are about 10 percent lower than those of intact females. The vitamin D3 levels of neutered male dogs is about 30 percent lower than those of intact males.
- The risk of getting cancer quadruples in dogs with lower stores of vitamin D3.
- A study confirms that 75 percent of all dogs and cats fed commercial dog food are deficient in vitamin D3.

For many years, I've suspected a vitamin D3 deficiency in both dogs and cats. I attribute the rise in cancer and many other diseases, in part, to this deficiency. I was delighted when VDI Laboratory started to test vitamin D3 levels in animals. Part of their studies dealt with several common dog breeds and found that the Golden Retriever, a breed that is very prone to cancer, has significantly lower D3 levels than most other breeds. Additional studies in the past have shown that low stores of vitamin D3 are associated with a wide variety of diseases in both dogs and cats in addition to cancer, including IBD, renal disease, heart disease, infections, feline tooth reabsorption, and hyperparathyroidism. Even a number of feline idiopathic hypercalcemias have resulted from D3 deficiency.

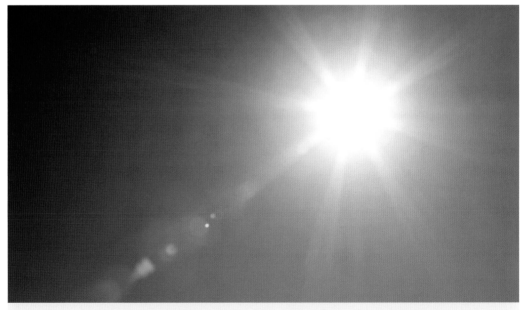

Unlike humans, who get vitamin D from the sun, dogs and cats rely on diet for sufficient levels of the vitamin.

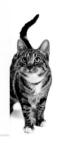

Vitamin D is a hormone, not a vitamin. It's biologically inert and must undergo two chemical reactions in the body to be activated. The first reaction occurs in the liver, and then a second reaction is needed; this occurs in the kidneys to create the active form of vitamin D3.

Dogs and cats get their D3 only from their diet. D3 is fat soluble, and, in pet foods, it comes from the fat of the meat product. If that's not enough, the manufacturers supplement with D3. But pets absorb their vitamin D3 precursor from meat fat much more readily than supplemental D3. Just like any other vitamin, cooking and heating can also destroy some of the vitamin D3.

The liver gets it all ready, but it's actually the kidneys that do the work to transform it into the active hormone. That's why cats with renal disease should be supplemented with D3. Of course, any pet with IBD will need supplemental D3.

IBD lowers the body's level of active D3 hormone. The typical conventional treatment for IBD is the oral administration of a steroid, such as prednisone. Steroid use upregulates the destruction of both forms of D3. It creates a situation that's a double-edged sword: low levels of D3 due to the IBD itself and increased destruction of D3 due to the steroid. Chronic IBD can lead to intestinal lymphosarcoma. It's not uncommon for cats with IBD to then get lymphosarcoma of the gut. Again, D3 deficiency increases cancer risk.

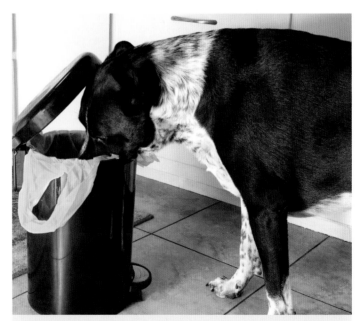

To successfully treat food-related problems, you must be aware of everything your dog eats, which means no garbage picking or counter surfing.

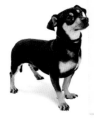

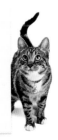

Did You Know?

Any kind of GI disorder will impair D3 absorption. The good news is that clinical evidence shows that correcting the vitamin D3 deficiency can improve the clinical signs of IBD. Because of the many variables, it's a good idea to have your pet tested for vitamin D3.

How to Treat Gastrointestinal Symptoms
Diarrhea

Pets with chronic bowel problems can have acute bouts of diarrhea over and over again, so it's important that pet owners know how to handle this problem quickly. The sooner you can help resolve your pet's acute diarrhea, the easier life will be for everyone in the household.

While getting into something in the garbage is a common cause of acute diarrhea in dogs, it's not the case with cats. Cats don't often get diarrhea from dietary indiscretions. Often, an acute bout of diarrhea in a cat is a sign of a more chronic intestinal problem. Both dogs and cats with acute diarrhea should be evaluated for possible intestinal-parasite infestation. If your dog or cat has both vomiting and diarrhea, it's time to get right to your veterinarian because these symptoms can be critical.

1. Pharmaceutical Drugs for Acute Diarrhea

Kaopectate®: Kaopectate is an over-the-counter drug available in drugstores and supermarkets. It contains a special mineral that absorbs the diarrhea-causing bacteria along with the toxins in the intestine. You can give your dog from 1 teaspoon to 1 tablespoon of Kaopectate every hour for three or four hours. It works best if given on the first day of the diarrhea.

Metronidazole: This drug must be dispensed or prescribed by your veterinarian. Oftentimes, giving just one pill when your pet first experiences diarrhea can nip the problem in the bud. Both dogs and cats can take metronidazole.

2. Homeopathic Remedies

Homeopathic remedies are ideal for acute diarrhea. Because they melt in the pet's mucous membranes and do not have to be swallowed, they are easy to administer, allowing you to rest the pet's digestive tract while treating him or her with some very effective medicine. It's a win-win situation.

Aloe 30c: This remedy is good for diarrhea with jellylike mucus in it. With this type of diarrhea, you may hear your pet's bowel rumbling, and he or she may need to eliminate with great urgency. You may give this remedy four times a day until the diarrhea clears up. Note: Mixing aloe 30c and podophyllum 30c and giving the mixture four times a day will help quickly alleviate most cases of uncomplicated diarrhea.

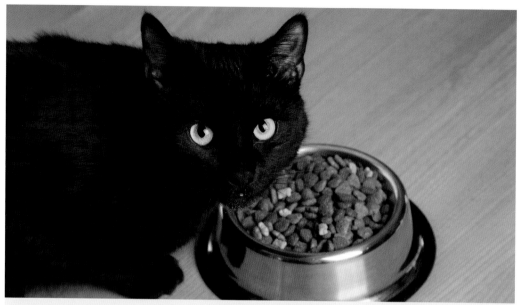

Isolating the problematic ingredient(s) in commercial food takes time and patience.

Arsenicum album 30c: This remedy is especially useful for cases of diarrhea accompanied by vomiting. The stool may have a very rank odor, and the pet may be restless. It is also a good remedy for dehydration. It should be given every hour or two, with the dosing reduced in frequency as improvement occurs. Keep dosing at least twice a day until the condition is well under control. See the vet if your pet does not respond to treatment.

China 30c: This remedy is important when your pet has lost a lot of fluid because it will help restore strength and maintain electrolyte balance. Give this remedy three times on the first day only.

Gallic acid: You can desensitize your pet to this problematic phenolic over a few months with a homeopathic preparation of gallic acid.

Merc cor 30c: This remedy is for diarrhea in which your pet strains to relieve him- or herself. Your pet may stay in the arch-backed position and go several times, producing diarrhea with mucus and a slimy appearance. There also may be spots of blood in the stool. Give this remedy three times a day to relieve symptoms, and I also recommend visiting the veterinarian for a checkup.

Nux vomica 30x: This is a good remedy to alleviate GI discomfort. Give once in the evening at bedtime.

Podophyllum 30c: This is a very good remedy for just about all cases of diarrhea, especially light brown or yellow diarrhea, which is very common in young nursing puppies. Give this remedy four times a day. After the stool becomes firm, reduce the frequency to twice a day for two to three days after the diarrhea has resolved.

3. Chinese Herbs

Po chai: You can find this common Chinese herb in most Chinese stores. This herb works wonderfully for dogs with acute diarrhea. It usually sold in sets of twelve small vials filled with tiny pellets. The dosage for a large dog is usually one vial three times a day. A small dog can get one half of a vial three times a day. Administer this herb until the diarrhea has fully cleared up, but do not continue use beyond that point.

4. Botanical Medicine

Carob powder: You can mix carob powder with water and give it to your pet. The recommended dosage is one-half to one teaspoon three times a day, depending on the size of the dog. You also can mix one teaspoon of slippery elm with teaspoon of carob powder and administer the two remedies together.

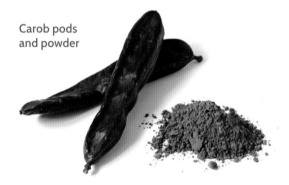

Carob pods and powder

Kudzu: In Japan and China, kudzu (kuzu) is the traditional medicine of choice for a host of digestive disorders. Kudzu's complex starch molecules enter the intestines and help restore health and stop diarrhea. Special antioxidants called *flavonoids* in the kudzu inhibit contractions of the smooth muscle tissue, stop cramping, and increase blood flow to the area. Kudzu also acts to thicken and regulate the intestinal contents and, thus, firm the stool. Kudzu is available in most health-food stores.

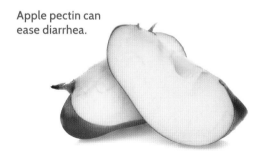

Apple pectin can ease diarrhea.

Pectin: Pectin, particularly apple pectin, has been a traditional treatment for acute diarrhea for decades. Pectin, as well as kaolin and bentonite clay, help stop diarrhea by latching onto the pathogens in the intestine and eliminating them. A veterinary over-the-counter product called Scour Aid contains

Kudzu Recipe to Stop Diarrhea

1 heaping teaspoon kudzu
3 tablespoons cold water
1 cup cold water
2 cups cooked white rice, cooked with chicken or beef bouillon cube
½ cup cooked chicken pieces, diced

Dissolve the kudzu in the 3 tablespoons of cold water. This mixture will be cloudy. Next, stir the dissolved kudzu into the rest of the cold water in a saucepan; the mixture will still be cloudy. Bring to a boil over medium heat and then reduce to low heat until the liquid looks translucent, stirring constantly to avoid lumping. Mix the liquid with the white rice and then add the diced chicken. Cool and serve.

both pectin and bentonite. The trick is to administer the product every two hours or so in the first stages of diarrhea. Small dogs weighing more than ten pounds can get one teaspoon, medium-sized dogs two teaspoons, and large dogs one tablespoon every two hours most of the day.

Slippery elm: This remedy, mixed with water, can be used with both dogs and cats. A small amount of powdered slippery elm bark in water forms a jellylike substance that you can administer to your pet to help slow the diarrhea. Typical dog dosage is one to two teaspoons three times a day, depending on the size of your dog, and one-half to one teaspoon for your cat.

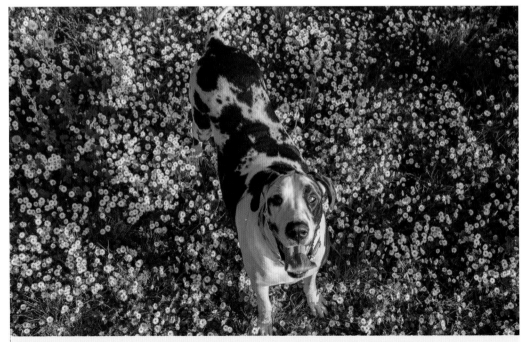

In some cases, environmental factors can exacerbate food-related symptoms.

More Antidiarrheal Recipes

Potato Stew

This recipe from Marty Goldstein, DVM, can be used for five to seven days to reduce diarrhea and loose stools, but not as a maintenance diet.

> White potatoes
> Sweet potatoes
> 1 slice turnip
> 1 leek
> Boiled chicken or beef

Boil equal parts white potatoes and sweet potatoes with the turnip and leek until cooked through. Mix in boiled meat for flavor.

Sweet Potato Stew

Sweet potatoes have a very calming effect on the intestines.

> 4 large sweet potatoes, baked or steamed
> 1 cup kefir or buttermilk or 3 hard-boiled eggs, mashed

Peel and mash sweet potatoes. Mix in other ingredients.

Combination Products

FullBucket® veterinary-strength supplements: These products, available in formulations for dogs and for cats, contain an enzyme blend, L-glutamine, prebiotics, and probiotics to help with diarrhea and loose stool. They have both dog and cat products.

Vetri-Science® Fast Balance GI Paste: This product for dogs contains mannan derived from the cell walls of yeast along with probiotics, enzymes, and B vitamins.

Vital Vities for Cats: This supplement by Deserving Pets contains prebiotics, probiotics, and L-glutamine and has proven to be helpful with chronic diarrhea in cats.

Vomiting

If your pet is vomiting repeatedly, he or she should see your veterinarian. Homeopathic remedies are the best treatment for mild cases of vomiting because they simply melt and are absorbed in the mouth.

Arsenicum album 30c: This is a good remedy for vomiting, especially when your pet has diarrhea along with vomiting. Administer it every hour until your pet's condition improves and then reduce the frequency of the doses as the problem starts to clear up; for example, give the remedy every hour for three doses, then every two hours for two doses, and then three times on the next day. Once the problem is resolved, stop the dosing altogether. The vomiting should begin to subside within three hours after starting the initial once-an-hour dosing. Of course, your pet should be resting his digestive tract.

Ipecac 30c: This homeopathic remedy can relieve the symptoms of vomiting. Ipecac is an excellent example of "like treats like"—as the straight compound, ipecac induces vomiting, but as a homeopathic remedy, it treats and relieves vomiting. This remedy can be given three times over a period of a day.

Constipation

It's not difficult to prevent or relieve simple constipation. In fact, many of the same things that work for people will also help your pet keep regular. If, however, the situation doesn't respond to early treatment and becomes chronic, it can be a signal of a larger problem.

Lack of roughage in the diet is the most common cause of simple constipation. This is particularly true of a diet very high in fat and meat and very low in roughage. Scan pet-food labels and purchase a food with ingredients such as blueberries, apples, beets, and herbs—all elements of good roughage.

The other basic causes of constipation are metabolic disorders or problems with certain organs. The colon is the part of the intestinal system that absorbs water. When the colon absorbs an abnormally high amount of water, stools

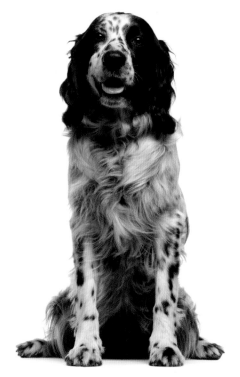

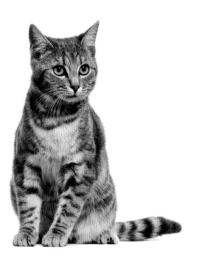

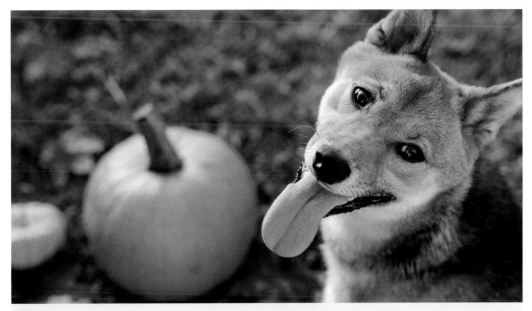

Pumpkin is your pet's friend when it comes to gastrointestinal problems.

become hard, dry, and difficult to pass. A few of the conditions affecting the colon and generating constipation through high absorption of water are kidney failure, heart failure, and diabetes.

You can give your pet homeopathic remedies and herbs in mild cases of constipation that are of short duration. If constipation persists for a period of time or for short durations with severity and straining, you should see your veterinarian.

An effective homeopathic remedy to help constipated pets is nux vomica 6x or 30x. It tones and detoxifies the digestive organs and is the first remedy to consider for constipation or sluggish bowels. Give this remedy three or four times a day for a few days and then reduce dosing to twice a day for one week.

Canned pumpkin is an effective addition to a pet's diet to help with constipation. It is an excellent source of fiber, and it works extremely well to prevent, correct, and counteract constipation. Additionally, be sure to keep your pet's water bowl full, promote exercise, and make sure his or her food has enough fiber and roughage.

Dietary fiber absorbs water in the intestines, making the stools larger, softer, and easier to pass. A sprinkle of bran cereal on your pet's food will add a healthy dose of dietary fiber. Psyllium husks and flaxseeds are also very high in fiber and good for the bowels. Make sure your pet is drinking plenty of water when you add fiber to his or her diet.

Add cooked vegetables and fresh fruit to your dog's diet or add some kitty greens or chlorophyll to your cat's diet. Add probiotics to your pets' food. Probiotics containing beneficial bacteria that make it to the gut, such as Probonix, available at Deserving Pets, help build the stool and encourage normal bowel movements.

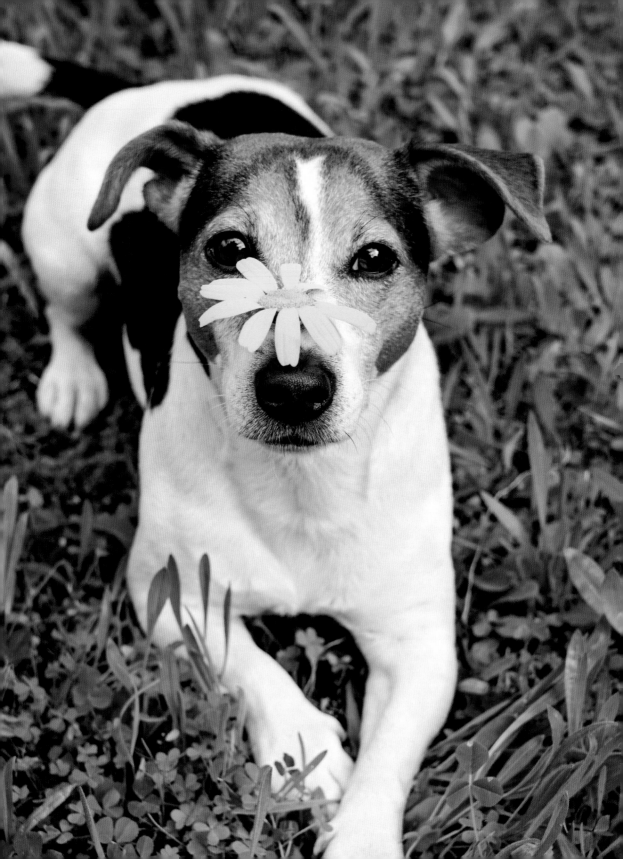

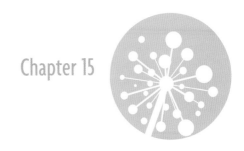

Chapter 15

Conventional versus Natural: Choosing Wisely

Our society can be extremely contradictory in its attitudes. For example, on one hand, we believe in saying no to drugs; on the other hand, we assiduously promote their use for all manner of ailments for people of all ages and for our pets. As long as they're manufactured by pharmaceutical companies, approved by the FDA, and, in many cases, prescribed by a doctor (or veterinarian), we consider them OK, even though we're well aware that many of them may have side effects.

I'm not trying to be insulting. It is well recognized that modern drugs have saved many a life. In fact, I use drugs when I deem it necessary in my practice and have saved lives as a result. If symptoms, such as an erratic heartbeat or high blood sugar, call for it, a doctor or veterinarian should prescribe the correct drug to help the sick individual compensate. No doubt about it, conventional medicine has come up with some impressive techniques and technologies for detecting and diagnosing disease.

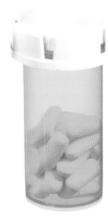

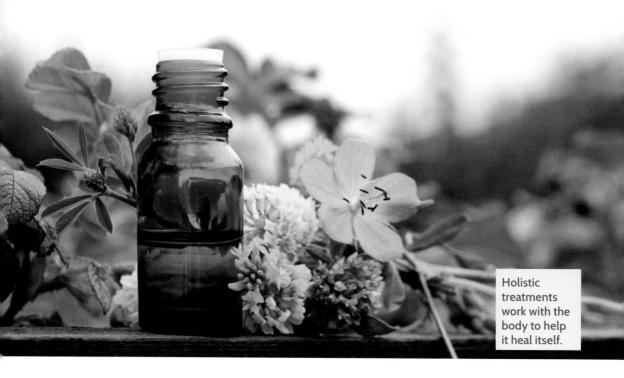

Holistic treatments work with the body to help it heal itself.

But pharmaceutical drugs work differently from holistic products. Pharmaceutical drugs typically alleviate symptoms. They rarely cure. At best, they buy time while the body heals. Taking a painkiller for a headache reduces the pain while the body works to heal itself. Someone suffering from migraines truly appreciates the relief. But the drug does not correct the actual problem or make the body more able. In all too many cases, the illness becomes chronic because the real source of the problem is never found and corrected.

Just treating symptoms can also curtail the body's ability to completely heal. The holistic approach assumes that the body is intelligent and that the symptoms are there for a reason. This is not to say that an illness or disease should be left untreated, assuming that your dog or cat will just heal on his or her own. Holistic treatments can be powerful tools that complement and enforce the body's innate ability to rebalance and restore itself, allowing the body to overcome the disease. Too many of us have long forgotten that the innate wisdom in the body, along with a little help from some holistic friends, can recreate true health.

Think of it this way: The dashboard of your automobile is equipped with a system of signals, or "symptoms." When the oil light goes on, it is a symptom that shows you that your engine needs oil. You could quickly suppress that symptom by finding the fuse box and pulling out the fuse that feeds your dashboard. Problem solved! The light is off, so everything is just fine. Or is it? We all know that this car will not last very long before the engine is destroyed because of the lack of oil. We can blissfully forget that we had a problem—until it is too late.

The use of drugs such as prednisolone, dexamethasone, cyclosporine, and others for allergic problems is basically following the same pattern. When you use these drugs to alleviate or suppress your pet's allergic symptoms, he or she will appear to quickly recover. Unless holistic intervention comes into play, your pet will likely become dependent on these drugs because his or her problems return soon after stopping the medications. Your pet winds up taking the drugs over and over again. Eventually, the owners realize that their pet has to be on these drugs every day because the drugs never cure the allergy; rather, they afford relief as the disease becomes more firmly embedded.

That said, while we all have to be informed about the effects of any conventional drug we give to our pets, we also need to be informed about the efficacy of holistic products that are commonly recommended for allergy problems. Here's the rub: Folks get on the Internet and start searching for some holistic product that will help their pet's itching or chronic diarrhea. If the product does not work, they may try another holistic fix that they find online. In the meantime, they're changing their pet's diet and wondering what is and what isn't really helping. If nothing works, they decide that they must resort to a lifetime of conventional drugs for allergies and/or food intolerances.

Supplements

I started creating supplements for dogs and cats because I wanted products of very high quality for my patients. Full understanding of the production process and the highest-quality ingredients are very important. For instance, the amount of a substance, such as cranberry, usually stated on the bottle in milligrams (mg), doesn't tell the whole story. Each sourced product has its own bioavailability. One cranberry source can be 70 percent bioavailable while another can be only 20 percent bioavailable, but the amount (mg) listed on the label will be the same in both cases. Often, products sold to doctors and veterinarians are made from higher-quality products because medical professionals won't keep buying the products if they are not seeing positive results.

You're going to learn how it all works: the processing, the oxidation, and the viability of the ingredients that work to help your pet. You'll learn how to find good products and evaluate your purchases; you may unknowingly be spending your hard-earned money on supplements that aren't what you think they are. You may surprised to find out how supplements can degrade during processing, while sitting on the shelf, and even after you open the bottle.

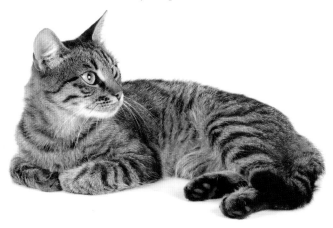

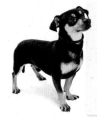
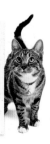

Most of us spend a great deal of time researching the supplements we give our dogs and cats. As a veterinarian, I'm no exception. We find ourselves reading labels and carefully comparing ingredients so we can give our best friends good-quality products but still live within our budgets.

Oxidation

Most of us think of oxygen as always being the good guy. When we breathe, it's "in with the good and out with the bad." And that's true for us. Yet, for vitamins and supplements, oxygen means death. Oxygen is the enemy of many natural plant compounds, which lose efficacy and potency rapidly when exposed to air.

Oxidation is a natural chemical process that occurs in fruit and vegetables. When their skin is broken, their cell walls and membranes rupture, allowing oxygen in. The nutrients react with the oxygen, incorporating the oxygen molecules into their own molecular structures. It's how fruit and vegetables spoil.

Peel a banana or cut an apple or avocado in half and watch what happens. It doesn't take long to see them start to turn brown. That's called surface oxidation.

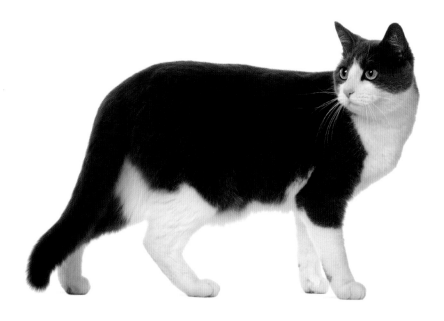

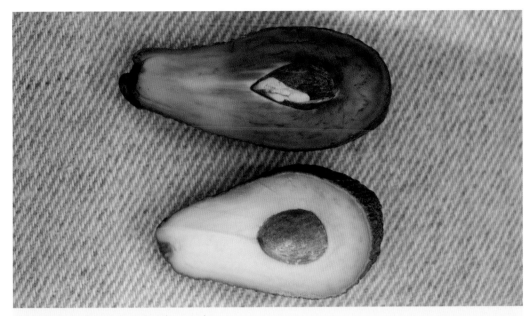

Ripe (bottom) versus oxidized avocado.

What's important for you to know is that when oxidation occurs, the fruit or vegetable loses most— or, more likely, *all*—of its nutritional value. The same oxidation that turns the apple brown after you cut it open works similar effects on your supplements. They're already in a very vulnerable form with their small surface area, which easily exposes the particles to air.

Many of us take B vitamins and may have experienced oxidation of supplements firsthand. The pills or tablets turn a brownish color and take on a rancid smell that increases over time. That's because they're oxidizing and losing their potency. The brown smelly capsules will have significantly fewer available B vitamins because they've simply been destroyed by exposure to oxygen.

Stability is an industry term that means "potency over time." Some vitamins lose their stability quickly, and some lose potency more slowly. I've joked that omega-3s lose all of their potency if you simply look at them the wrong way. They are so sensitive to light, air, and heat that most omega-3 supplements are not worth purchasing.

This brings me to the other enemies of nutritional value: light and heat. Oxygen, light, and heat all contribute to the destruction of the products we purchase.

Along with Omega 3s and B vitamins, there are other vitamins that degrade and oxidize when exposed to heat, light, and oxygen. For example, just as fruit darkens with exposure to oxygen, vitamin C will turn a darker color after you open the bottle repeatedly.

The fat-soluble vitamins A and E are particularly prone to oxidation and they lose their nutritional value over a relatively short period of time. For example, the pink color in salmon due to carotenoids (a form of vitamin A) will disappear due to oxidation.

Omega-3s: Fishing for the Truth

While omega-6 fatty acids are plentiful in our pets' diets, regardless of what they eat, omega-3s are not. Because omega-3s are fragile and break down quickly in the presence of heat, air, or light, they are lacking in both the commercial and fresh foods that we tend to feed. Remember, pet foods are highly heated and processed, and omega-3s cannot survive the process. While pet food labels may state that omega-3 and omega-6 essential fatty acids have been added to the food, even if they are added after processing, the reality is that the food is deficient in omega-3s due to unavoidable exposure to air and light. Omega-3s are notorious for their lack of stability.

Supplement companies measure their ingredient levels with a Certificate of Analysis (COA) *before* the processing begins. The supplement goes into gel capsules, most of which are permeable to air, and then placed in plastic containers that are not airtight. Or they may go into pump bottles, which add air back into the bottles with every pump. Then the product sits on the shelf in the store or in your cupboard and, at the end of the day, you wind up with negligible amounts of the product you purchased. The bottom line is that what is stated on the label surely does not reflect the reduced value of the product.

I no longer recommend fish oil as a source of omega-3s. Fish oils turn rancid very easily, which can cause them to become toxic. The pungent odor or "off" flavor, along with gel-capsule discoloration, tells the story. However, fish oils often contain flavors to mask the odor of oxidation and make them more palatable. Another problem is that dogs and cats given fish oil capsules every day can become allergic to fish because of the continual exposure.

The only fish oils I ever recommend are made from wild-caught anchovies, sardines, and mackerel from the deep, clear waters of the Pacific in South America followed by triple distillation in Norway. This prevents contamination with mercury, PCBs, dioxins, dieldrin, and toxaphene—all poisons in one way or another. I'll just add to this how hard it can be to find out whether the product is produced this way and is free of these toxins either by reading the label or contacting the company directly.

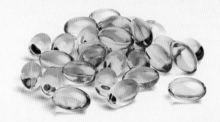

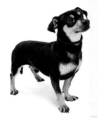
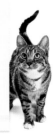

Fruits and vegetables are most attractive to humans and animals when they are perfectly ripe, which is also when they are the most nutritious. Once they spoil and become putrid, we're instead repulsed by the same food. There are no health benefits associated with eating rotten produce, and the same goes for our supplements—except that supplements may have flavor added to mask the oxidation or encapsulation to hide the odor.

Preserving Ingredients

Some companies, in an effort to avoid degradation of their products, have gone to great lengths to protect their precious ingredients.

Resveratrol is enjoying a boost in popularity these days. It's extracted from seventy different plants, including pomegranates, blueberries, and many types of nuts. Yet resveratrol, once exposed to air, light, and heat, will degrade rapidly. This decreases its health benefits, because only trans-resveratrol activates the SiRT1 gene that repairs DNA. Most supplements sold today contain high amounts of degraded resveratrol, making them mostly ineffective.

At one point, I began researching resveratrol for its potential ability to control canine lymphoma. People were giving huge doses of a resveratrol product from China with few results, but much smaller doses from one particular company had some very promising outcomes. Why would this be? The answer to this question again emphasizes the importance of getting quality products that are not oxidized on the assembly line or when sitting around on the stockroom floor.

When I called the company, once again on my mission, the representative told me in passing that they used a major pharmaceutical company to encapsulate the product. I asked him why, and he explained that the pharmaceutical company had inherited an unusual piece of equipment when they purchased another company. The equipment

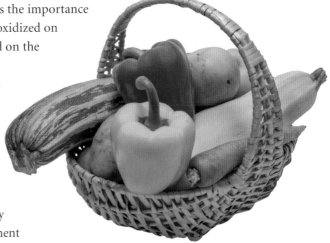

pumped all the air out of the encapsulation chamber and filled it with nitrogen. The product was pumped in without exposure to air, light, or heat. Each capsule was impermeable to air and light, and each was individually blister-packed. With this method, the customer was getting exactly what was stated on the label of the product, unlike with other resveratrol products.

Some companies use microencapsulation to stabilize their products. Microencapsulation is a process in which very tiny particles are surrounded by a coating to prevent their degradation and increase their stability by isolating vitamins and nutrients from the deteriorating effects of oxygen. Some companies microencapsulate all of the ingredients in their supplements to preserve their stability.

For example, Deserving Pets makes a canine supplement (Canine Everyday Essentials) and a feline supplement (Vital Vities for Cats) that contain antioxidants, vitamins, minerals, superfoods, and phytochemicals that are all human-grade and completely balanced with generous doses of all ingredients. Every single ingredient is coated by microencapsulation to prevent oxidation and keep the ingredients pure and fresh.

The marketplace is filled with exciting new products that have great promise. Yet, to fulfill that promise, the bottle actually has to contain what's stated on the label. Shop carefully for all of your pet's supplements.

I recommend that, unless your pet's supplements are protected from degradation, you buy supplements in glass bottles (which, unlike plastic, are impervious to air); store them, tightly capped, in the refrigerator; and try to minimize their exposure to air.

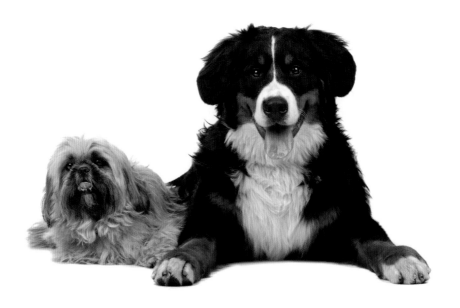

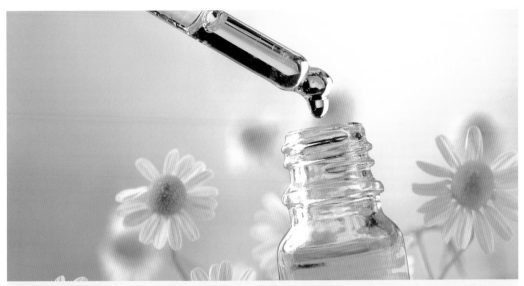

Effective supplements come from natural sources, such as fruits, vegetables, herbs, and other plants.

What Really Works?

Which supplements actually work for itching pets? Following are some of the products that I recommend. Keep in mind that each pet is an individual and will respond better to some supplements than others. The only way to know is to try.

Antronex®: Bovine liver fat extract and calcium work together to support healthy immune processes in dogs and cats. I especially like this product for itchy cats because cats often seem to like the taste of the tablets and will eat them with no problem.

Beta-sitosterol plant sterols: Formulated to help regulate cholesterol, this natural plant sterol acts like a natural anti-inflammatory with steroid-like calming properties to relieve itching without the steroids. Beta-Thym™ is a natural beta-sitosterol formulation that acts like a corticosteroid in a natural form. It also contains thymus extract and ornithine to support the immune system.

HistoPlex-AB®: This is a blend of herbs that supports respiratory and immune function to help pets better cope with the onset of allergies, resulting in less severe reactions.

Phytosterols: Plant phytosterols, which are natural components of plants such as vegetables and grains, help support healthy immune systems and healthy cholesterol levels already within the normal range. The three main phytosterols in phytosterol complex are beta-sitosterol, campesterol, and stigmasterol. They are natural, safe, and derived entirely from plant sources.

Quercetin: This natural solution lives in the peels of many fruits and vegetables. It's a flavonoid, meaning that it is a plant-based compound with powerful antioxidant, anti-inflammatory, and antihistamine characteristics. Because histamine is a major player in itchy skin, quercitin can be very helpful in "turning off" histamine production and moderate inflammation. For this reason, many have coined it "nature's Benadryl®."

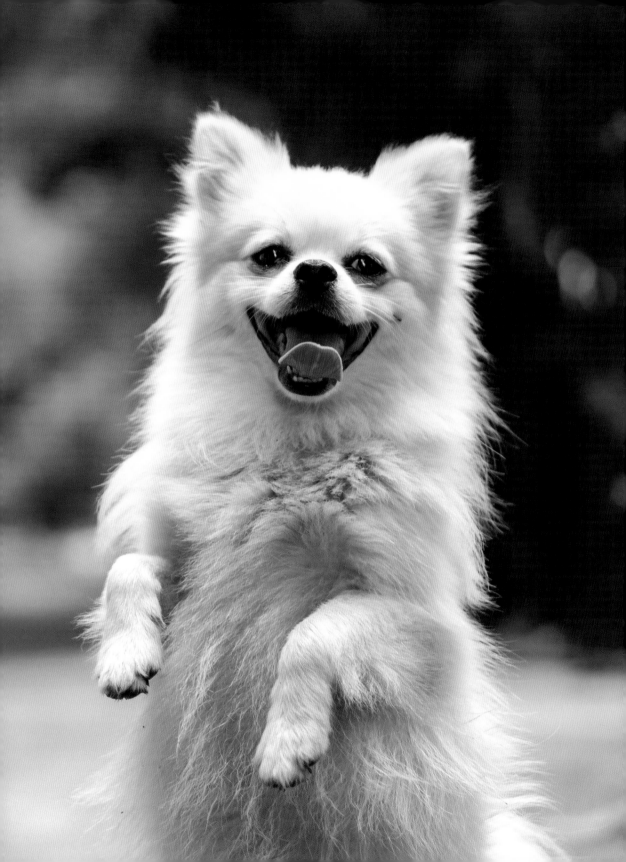

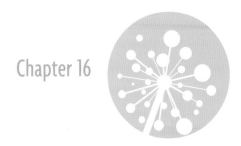

Chapter 16

Allergy Elimination: Getting Rid of Allergies and Sensitivities for Good

---

*T*he most efficient solution to the allergy problem in our pets would be to fix their faulty immune systems—the computers that have, so to speak, gone awry in our pets' bodies. And that's why holistic solutions, particularly Allergy Elimination 4 Pets, can be especially effective. An easy way to understand Allergy Elimination 4 Pets is to make the parallel example of doing a virus search on your computer to clean up the glitches. Allergy Elimination 4 Pets works to clean up and straighten out your pet's computer.

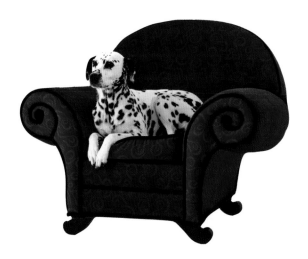

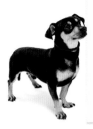
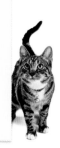
My first allergy-elimination class was on something called Nambudripad's Allergy Elimination Technique (NAET®). Dr. Nambudripad's method is where it all started. Devi Nambudripad, PhD, MD, DC, LAc, the founder of NAET, had been very ill with allergies all her life. I wouldn't be exaggerating too much if I said that she was allergic to almost everything under the sun. She lived exclusively on polished white rice and broccoli. One day, she decided to "take a walk on the wild side" and have a carrot. She started to pass out, so gave herself an acupuncture treatment to keep herself from going into shock. She fell asleep and awoke forty-five minutes later with a feeling of complete well-being.

She researched her experience and discovered that when you hold an allergenic substance within your body's electromagnetic field while receiving a treatment for the adverse allergic reaction, your body's systems somehow self-correct. The body recognizes the electromagnetic signature of the

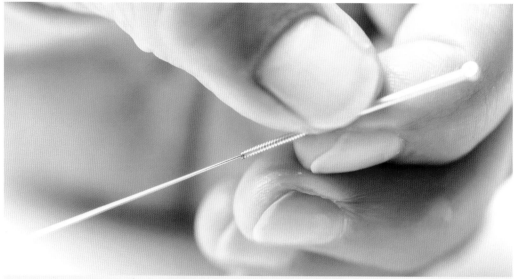

Acupuncture principles are at the core of NAET.

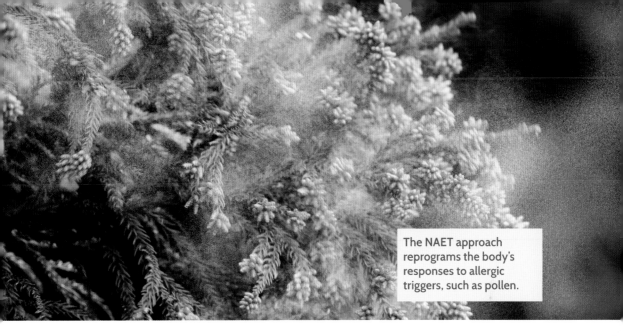

The NAET approach reprograms the body's responses to allergic triggers, such as pollen.

substance while being encouraged, by the stimulation of acupuncture points, to start the process of healing, repairing, correcting, and harmonizing. Whatever the reason—karma, kismet, or serendipity—the manner in which Dr. Nambudripad discovered this very workable technique was indeed fortuitous.

The genius of Dr. Nambudripad's approach is that it takes the allergy out of any substance and turns the allergic body into the allergy-free body. The brain, or, more accurately, the autonomic nervous system, reinterprets what it used to think of as an allergen and instead begins to see it in a new light as a harmless, acceptable substance. That's how your pet's body should react in a healthy state.

It's interesting to note that when we enter the realm of energetic holistic medicine, we leave the field of biology and enter the field of physics. Every day, new research in physics challenges old beliefs about how the body works and heals. Even though the Chinese recognized energy pathways (called *acupuncture meridians*) more than 6,000 years ago, it has taken the advent of new scientific methodologies to recognize how changes in energy fields affect and determine health.

The autonomic nervous system plays an integral role in recognizing what the body's computer has deemed enemies. It then calls the immune system into action to defend the body against the enemy.

Allergy Treatment at Home

Practitioners expanded upon NAET to create diverse allergy-elimination programs. Using the knowledge from many diverse courses and my extensive clinical experience, I refined them all into the easy-to-do-at-home Allergy Elimination 4 Pets.

Applied Kinesiology

In 1964, an American chiropractor named George Goodheart began to use muscle testing to evaluate muscle function, posture, and general body imbalances. His continued research led him to formulate applied kinesiology (AK). Many professionals, including dentists, medical doctors, osteopaths, naturopaths, psychologists, and veterinarians have been trained in and utilize AK in their practices.

The International College of Applied Kinesiology (ICAK) seeks to promote the advancement of AK. Founded in 1973, it now has chapters in the United States, Canada, Europe, Japan, Russia, and Australasia. The organization awards certification to practice AK. Applicants must have more than three hundred hours of instruction and pass several proficiency examinations.

Muscle response testing (MRT) is a specific technique, evolving from AK, and it is used as an effective and versatile tool for detecting various imbalances in the body, including allergic substances and food and environmental sensitivities and intolerances. This exciting aspect of kinesiology is sometimes referred to as *specialized kinesiology*.

Allergy-elimination techniques such as NAET correct the autonomic nervous system's perception of the allergic substance so it is no longer perceived as a threat. It all happens within the realm of physics on an energetic level, and it translates into physical healing. Each treatment teaches your pet's body that an allergen is a friend rather than an enemy.

Over the years, many practitioners have modified NAET, and it is referred to by several different names. The technique I have designed and use is called Allergy Elimination 4 Pets.

The typical scenario of the owner of an allergic pet is a path of avoidance—and it's a lifelong job. It simply doesn't have to be that way. If you've been dealing with your pet's allergies for years, it may be hard for you to believe that there exists an allergy-elimination technique that transforms an allergic pet into a nonallergic pet. It may seem too good to be true that you can turn your pet's chronic problems around, but it happens all the time.

After first identifying a pet's allergy triggers through muscle response testing (applied kinesiology), I work with the pet owner to correct the blockages or imbalances. I do this by correcting the immune system's misperception of the allergen, which, in effect, enables the body to heal itself by restoring the unrestricted flow of energy. Think of it as corrective reprogramming.

It all happens within the realm of physics on an energetic level and translates into physical healing. A specific program is created for each pet. The energetic resonance of each allergen combination that your pet needs is placed in a vial. The vial containing the allergen is placed directly on the animal, and specific acupuncture points on the body are lightly stimulated. This

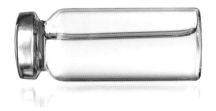

readjusts the autonomic nervous system's perception of the substance, and the allergic reaction to the substance is eliminated. It may be amazing to learn that something so simple can work so well, but the proof is in the rewarding results.

The first step is identifying the substances to which the patient is allergic. In the first comprehensive assessment, approximately 500 vials specifically designed for this purpose are checked using muscle response testing. So what exactly is muscle response testing?

Professional medical doctors, chiropractors, acupuncturists, and veterinarians use muscle response testing, or applied kinesiology, to determine exactly what a person or pet is allergic to. The inventor of applied kinesiology is George Goodheart, Jr., DC, a Detroit chiropractor. After his first seminar in 1974, many other practitioners began using the technique with great success to determine the causes of problems that had previously seemed to defy diagnosis.

In the decades since then, this method of testing for the causes of various conditions has blossomed into a major diagnostic art, with many more medical professionals, including veterinarians, adopting it in their practices. (The book *Your Body Doesn't Lie* by John Diamond, MD, is an excellent source of information on the subject.) Allergy-elimination treatments that have stemmed from NAET do not only relieve the symptoms but also correct the inappropriate response. These treatments have helped many pet owners and their best friends live happier and fuller lives.

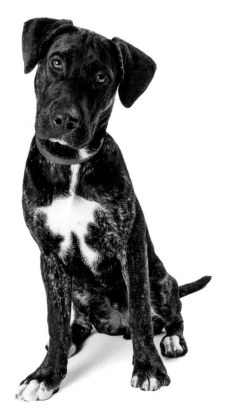

I've been practicing different varieties of allergy elimination techniques for so many years, and, with my extensive clinical experience, I pretty well know what vials need to be used with most dogs or cats with allergies. That's good news for you and your pet because my protocol has been tested over time with many, many patients.

After I've identified the allergens through muscle response testing, I decide in which order to treat the allergens and create a program for the patient. I then mail the vials to the pet owner along with clear instructions on how to gently massage easy-to-find acupuncture points (cats particularly appreciate this!) and carry out the treatment in the comfort of his or her home.

More about Nellie

Nellie, a wonderful Golden Retriever who is a patient of mine, can testify to the curative powers of these healing methods. Here, in her own words (with her owners' help in providing a translation from "caninese") is her story: one dog's odyssey through the medical system in search of allergy relief.

When I was a little over a year old, I began doing things like licking my paws and running my face along the carpets. My owners, who are very attentive, took me right to a veterinarian, who diagnosed my problem as an allergy and started me on a course of daily steroids. But even on a really high dose, I didn't improve. We then tried antihistamines, but they didn't help, either. I was then tested for a thyroid condition, and prescribed another drug, called levothyroxine, along with more steroids and antibiotics, which seemed to work for a while. But the steroids I was taking caused me to drink water constantly, so my owners tried to cut back on them, and I got very itchy again.

A year later, my owners decided to try another veterinarian. I went home with a new steroid and more antibiotics. Soon, my chest hair was gone and my skin had become thick and greasy. My paws didn't look so good, either. We then went to a third doctor, who took a blood sample from me and sent it away to determine what exactly I was allergic to. The doctor gave my owners a serum that they injected under my skin every week. The vet told my owners that it would take at least nine months for the injections to work, but I still was no better after more than a year.

The next stop was a veterinary school hospital (my owners spared no expense to try to get me healthy), where I was given a skin test for allergies. From this test, doctors developed another serum. With new serum, antibiotics, and antihistamines, I just kept getting worse.

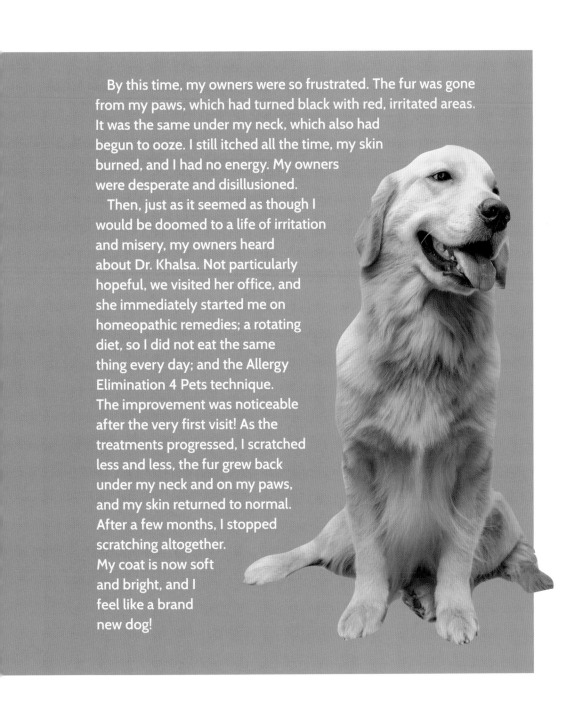

By this time, my owners were so frustrated. The fur was gone from my paws, which had turned black with red, irritated areas. It was the same under my neck, which also had begun to ooze. I still itched all the time, my skin burned, and I had no energy. My owners were desperate and disillusioned.

Then, just as it seemed as though I would be doomed to a life of irritation and misery, my owners heard about Dr. Khalsa. Not particularly hopeful, we visited her office, and she immediately started me on homeopathic remedies; a rotating diet, so I did not eat the same thing every day; and the Allergy Elimination 4 Pets technique. The improvement was noticeable after the very first visit! As the treatments progressed, I scratched less and less, the fur grew back under my neck and on my paws, and my skin returned to normal. After a few months, I stopped scratching altogether. My coat is now soft and bright, and I feel like a brand new dog!

With Allergy Elimination 4 Pets, I use glass vials containing the energetic resonance of individual or combined allergens that are recognized by your pet's autonomic nervous system on an energetic level. These vials are glass because the energetic resonances can get through glass, but not plastic. It's pretty incredible. After years and years of watching the so-called miracles occur, I'm still very impressed.

Often, people contact me through my website (*www.doctordeva.com*) and request a consultation. The first thing I do is review the pet's records carefully and make sure that there are no "allergy impersonators" in play. If Allergy Elimination 4 Pets is the indicated treatment, I do muscle response testing for allergens and sensitivities and prepare a program for the individual pet. Dogs and cats with IBD mostly require corrections to foods and phenolics, along with the mycoplasmas that are indicated in Crohn's disease. Dogs and cats with itching problems always need corrections to foods along with the correctly chosen environmental allergens.

You should know that there is an order and a specific combination strategy that pets do well with. You see, we can't overwhelm your pet with too much too fast—it just doesn't work . That's why you can only use a particular number of items in each treatment. For example, you can't do a treatment for your pet's commercial kibble all at once, because the food has many different components as well as phenolics, as we discussed previously.

DIY

For those pet owners who don't have a holistic practitioner available and who don't contact me for a consultation, I've developed a prepared set of vials that covers a lot of ground. That said, there are

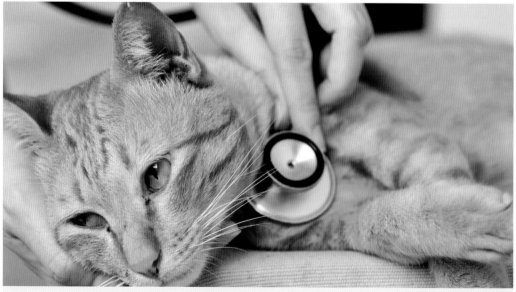

Your vet will start with a thorough exam before prescribing a plan for allergy treatment.

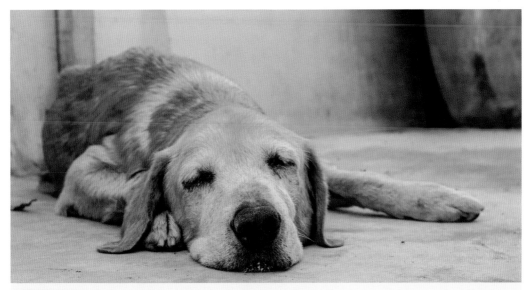
Allergies affect a pet's energy and activity levels.

triggers that are not included in this kit. For instance, few people have wool carpets, but wool can become quite the culprit for pets who are on the carpet all the time. See Appendix III (page 212) for specific information about the vial kit.

Autoimmune Diseases: When the Body "Chases Its Own Tail"

Malfunctions of the body's immune system that represent more serious health problems for both pets and people are known as *autoimmune diseases*. As with allergies, these afflictions result from the immune system responding to "false alarms" and zeroing in on the wrong target. When this happens, the consequences can include serious diseases, such as lupus, which produces generalized and systemic malaise and extreme sensitivity to sunlight; blood diseases that attack and destroy red blood cells or platelets; and conditions that affect the kidneys, causing them to lose protein.

Why Does the Immune System Behave This Way?

Some experts believe that when an autoimmune response occurs, the immune system is actually chasing down an elusive invader hiding in the tissues. And, in fact, research has given this added credence, showing that tiny pathogens called mycoplasmas—the smallest microorganisms known to science that are able to self-replicate—can evade the immune system in this manner. These amorphous little creatures can change their shapes to appear and disappear at will, concealing themselves within body tissues and fluids, and are very difficult to track down. For instance, because they don't carry any antigenic markers that the immune system can recognize and attack, their presence isn't revealed by blood tests used to detect disease. They can also reemerge from their hiding places inside cells once the coast is clear.

> ## Three Things to Remember
> 1. Your pet is subject to the same types of immune-system-related disorders as you are, ranging from annoying allergies to crippling, possibly life-threatening, autoimmune diseases.
> 2. Conventional treatments are likely to offer only limited, if any, relief and may produce side effects.
> 3. There are safe, proven noninvasive holistic alternative treatments that can bring your pet the kind of permanent relief that drugs seldom provide.

Other pathogens, such as *Borrelia*—the bacterium that causes Lyme disease—can invade tissues and create cysts that can produce potent toxins, causing an autoimmune response. Routine antibiotics unfortunately won't destroy these cysts, which can remain long after Lyme disease symptoms are thought to be under control. To make matters worse, Lyme-causing *Borrelia* and mycoplasmas often work together as coinfections for a kind of double whammy. And the fact that ticks can carry both pathogens completes this rather dismal picture.

What makes mycoplasmas particularly pernicious is their ability to move into cells and steal the protein, fats, and vitamins that they need to survive but lack the genes to make themselves. Sometimes described as *parasitic bacteria*, mycoplasmas have been known to squeeze through filters used to maintain sterility in hospitals and laboratories and to have been sources of contamination in everything from important experiments to routine vaccinations. They are believed to play a major role in such afflictions as osteoarthritis, rheumatoid arthritis, Crohn's disease, IBD, and chronic fatigue syndrome, as well as autoimmune diseases that cause a degenerative erosion of the fatty myelin sheaths that protect and insulate nerve fibers, such as multiple sclerosis. They have also been linked to lymphoma and implicated in the development of other cancers. Darryl See, MD, and Ferre Akbarpour, MD, of the Orange County Immune Institute in Huntington Beach, California, have determined that almost 90 percent of certain late-stage cancer patients are infected with pathogenic mycoplasmas, which are believed to contribute to cancer formation by releasing cell-damaging free radicals.

To conceal themselves in your pet's body, mycoplasmas use molecular mimicry to disguise themselves so that they resemble the host cells, for instance, by incorporating the cells' surface material into their own jellylike surfaces. This is what may confuse the immune system into attacking the body's own tissues, sort of like a fox hunter on a horse who chops up the flower beds, landscape, and shrubbery in the pursuit of his quarry.

According to this theory, if the mycoplasma hides, for example, in a dog's joint tissue, the dog's immune system will attempt to destroy the mycoplasma and will fail, causing a lot of inflammation, which eventually develops into arthritis.

Barkley's Story

by Barkley's owner

Barkley, my male Rhodesian Ridgeback, didn't seem to be walking right when he was about six months of age. The veterinarian examined him and found that many of the joints in his legs were swollen, hot, and painful. Tests showed he had rheumatoid arthritis. The vet told me that Barkley could not be cured and that he would have to be on medication to suppress his immune system for the rest of his life. I was devastated.

Even on the medication, Barkley was lame and sore and didn't seem to enjoy life. It broke my heart that he did not experience a real "puppyhood."

I heard about Dr. Khalsa, and I called her. Amazingly, she felt very positive about treatment. She sent me some vials, and I treated him at home; within a month, I had a normal dog. We weaned him off his medications, and Dr. Khalsa sent me Double Helix Water to put in his drinking water every day, which was holistic and natural and—I keep saying amazingly because it really was—he became a normal, healthy dog with normal blood tests, and the problem was actually cured. I can't thank Dr. Khalsa enough for her compassion and kindness and for all the knowledge she has up her sleeve. It was so effortless that it was almost fun, and I get to have a healthy, normal dog. Better yet, Barkley now has a quality life.

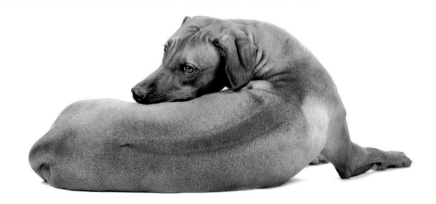

One thing we can say with some degree of certainty is that a body with a less-than-optimal pH, as described in Chapter 11, is the ideal habitat for these pathogens. This is yet another reason why a healthy, well-balanced diet is so important to your pet's well-being.

More on JMT

Once mycoplasmas were identified as the prime suspects, or external pathogenic factors (EPFs) in triggering a host of ailments, holistic practitioners Dr. Carolyn Jaffe, LAc, DOM, NMD, and Judith Mellor, RN, developed a revolutionary technique for reprogramming the immune system that was laying waste to the body's tissues in its attempt to rout out the invaders. The Jaffe-Mellor Technique® (JMT) has established an impressive track record of successfully eliminating the symptoms of osteoarthritis and other degenerative bone disorders and significantly reducing the pain and other symptoms that accompany Lyme disease, rheumatoid arthritis, lupus, fibromyalgia, Crohn's disease, multiple sclerosis, muscular dystrophy, and other autoimmune ailments.

What the pair determined is that disorders caused by EPFs are far more common than previously imagined. When the autonomous nervous system is alerted to the presence of these

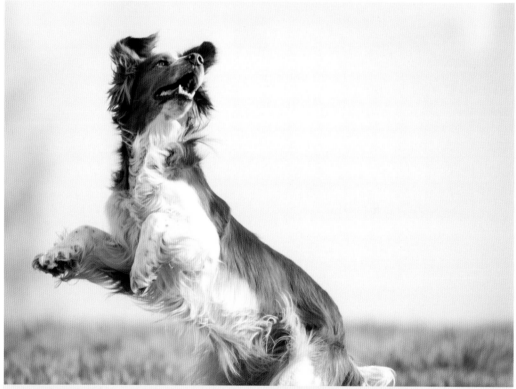

When his body is rebalanced, your pet can get back to his lively, fun self.

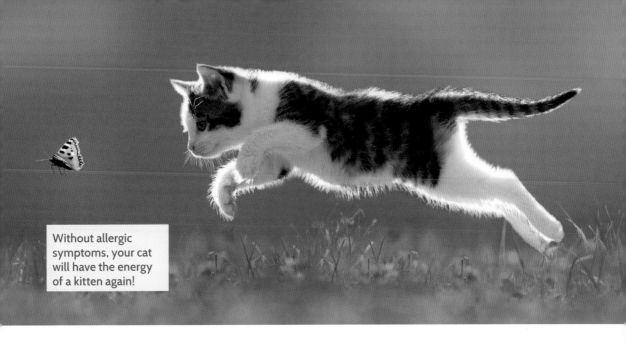

Without allergic symptoms, your cat will have the energy of a kitten again!

stealth invaders, it signals the immune system to go on a search-and-destroy mission wherever the pathogens have colonized in the body, be it joints, cartilage, muscles, bone tissue, kidneys, liver, skin, or the nervous system itself. Because there are so many different components comprising the immune system, it is as if the Army, Navy, Marines, and Air Force all launched simultaneous strikes with a multitude of weapons, leaving devastated towns and villages in their wake.

To correct this situation, JMT utilizes a combination of holistic therapies to restore harmony to the body and its magnetic field, correct any energetic imbalance, and recharge the brain and nervous system to eliminate flawed programming. This includes an advanced form of muscle-resistance testing to determine the presence of pathogens, and the use of acupressure or a laser to activate the acupuncture points. The result is reprogramming of the immune system and deactivation and neutralization of the pathogen. Finally, the damaged tissues are taught to repair themselves and the body reeducated to produce normal cartilage.

To administer this treatment to your pet, I ascertain what vials are needed and determine what needs to be corrected. The procedure itself involves placing the appropriate energetic resonance of the pathogen on your pet, after which you will be trained to apply acupressure to certain areas to balance the energy throughout his or her body. The treatments are risk-free, noninvasive, and painless, and the pet often feels relief after only one or two sessions. However, several different treatments may be required to correct and repair each "layer" of the disease. After the pathogen is deactivated in this manner, the damaged tissue will finally begin to heal. I know it may sound strange and confusing to many people, and perhaps even too good to be true, but I can assure you from personal experience that it works like a charm!

I have used this technique for a number of years in my practice with truly miraculous results. I have found it to be one of the most exciting therapies available in the field of holistic medicine and an appropriate way to treat a wide range of severe illnesses in pets.

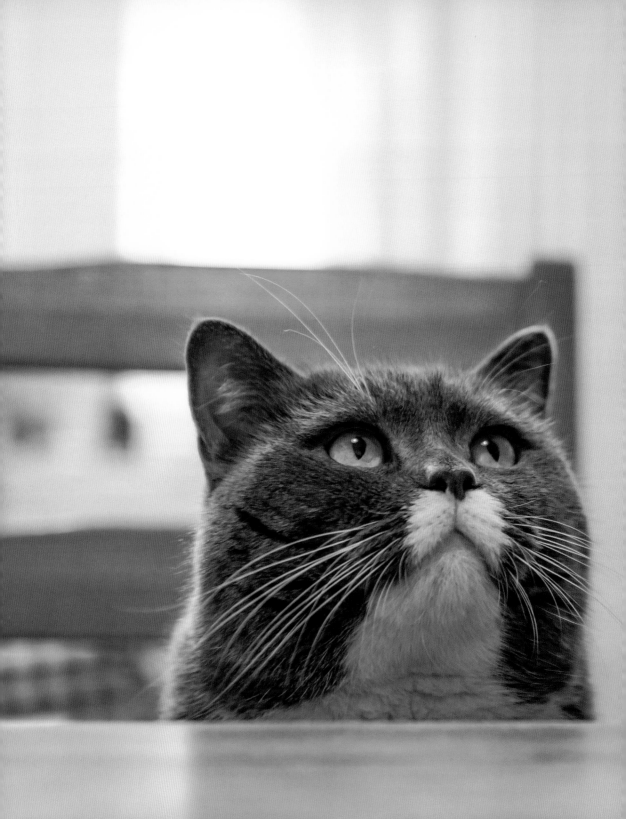

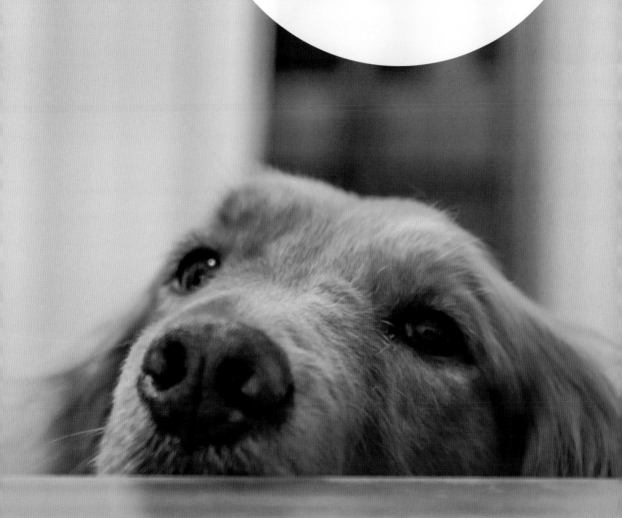

Part III
Finding Food that Works

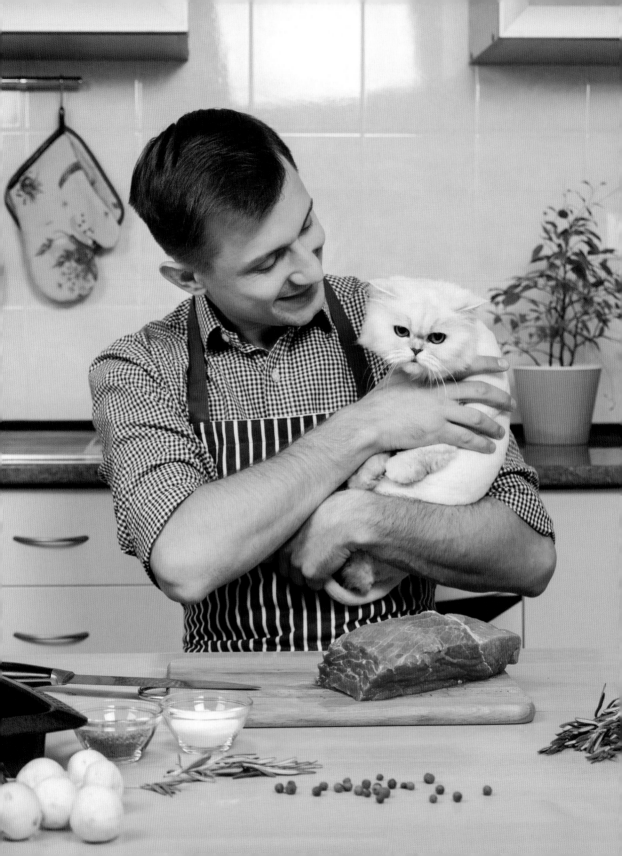

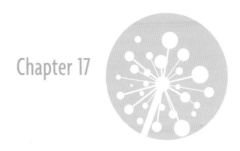

Chapter 17

Feeding Furry Friends: Nutrition Advice and Recipes

Our plan is to cure our pets of food allergies and intolerances because they are major causes of skin and gastrointestinal distress. Choosing what to feed an allergic pet often causes stress and confusion.

Many people who want to serve homemade food to their pets worry about what to cook. Many other concerned owners just don't have time to make homemade meals for their pets. If you choose to feed a commercial diet, there are many suitable formulas that have novel proteins along with other novel ingredients. There is

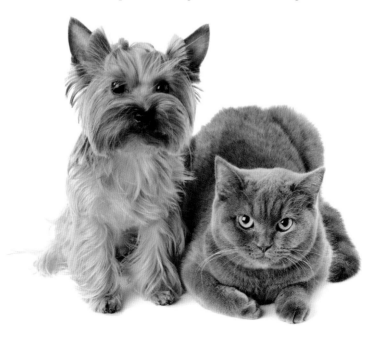

also the option of combining the best of both worlds, for example, serving a commercial food in the morning and then a homemade meal in the evening.

Once your dog or cat is free of food-related symptoms, you will no longer have to feed special diets and novel proteins. If you vary your pet's diet, add a good supplement, and feed proper portions and proportions, you'll have all of the bases covered. And that's exactly we are going to discuss now.

Feeding Your Allergic Dog
Meals: How Big?

How big should a dog's meals be? You can refer to the chart below as a basic guideline for determining daily portions for your dog. It's best to keep a watchful eye on your dog's weight, appetite, and body condition and alter the amounts accordingly.

Weight and Portions

Pounds	Amount of dry food a day (if you feed only dry food)	Amount of cooked food a day (if you feed only cooked food)
15	1½ cups	1½–2 cups
25	2 cups	1¾–2½ cups
40	3 cups	2½–3½ cups
60	4 cups	4–4½ cups
100	6 cups	5–7 cups

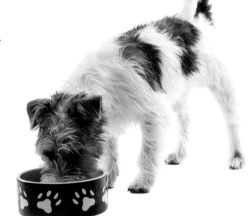

Dogs are really a lot like we are in this respect. There are people who eat whatever they want and maintain picture-perfect figures, and those who stay heavy despite eating well. Also like humans, dogs tend to gain weight more easily as they age. Additionally, some people and dogs are physically active, while others are more sedentary. The combination of metabolism, age, and lifestyle should strongly influence how much you feed your dog.

Before changing your dog's diet, weigh him to get a reference point. He may lose some weight initially on this diet because of its roughage and fiber content. As his weight readjusts, you may find that you need to feed him more or less to maintain a desirable weight. The chart will provide you with guidelines for where to start.

> ## Caution!
> The following items are harmful to dogs: citrus fruit, grapes, raisins, xylitol (artificial sweetener), onions, strawberries, yeast dough, coffee, tea, cola, and chocolate.

Remember that a dog does not have to eat his entire daily portion in one meal. Dogs are pack animals, and they like to eat when their families do, which is usually in the morning and evening—breakfast and dinner. A 40-pound dog can have, for example, 1¼ cups of oatmeal and some goat yogurt or a "meal in a muffin" (such as the one on page 195) in the morning and then 2¼ cups of one of the stews you'll find in the recipe section for dinner.

Variety: The Spice of Life

Variety in a dog's diet ensures balance. You can easily mix and match vegetables and fruits, carbohydrates, and protein sources, and it can be fun to do as you come up with new ideas for nutritious combinations. There are always some exceptions, but our dogs seem to like whatever we prepare for them—and we don't have to be professional chefs to put together delicious and healthy meals.

My rule of thumb, which holistic veterinarians have used for years, is to create meals with proportions of one-third carbohydrates, one-third protein, and one-third vegetables and add a little olive oil. I recommend varying your dog's diet, but you can make some big pots of your ingredient choices and, after using them up, move on to a new combination.

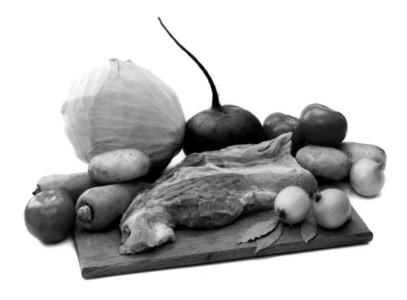

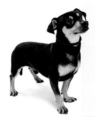
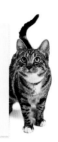

Did You Know?

Unlike powdered bone meal, green vegetables contain easily absorbable water-soluble calcium. Be generous with the greens in your dog's meals.

Here are a few tips:

- You must cook fish and pork, but you can serve beef, venison, and chicken either cooked, raw, or lightly seared.
- You can cook grains, such as quinoa, millet, and brown rice, in large quantities and use them with each recipe or freeze until needed.
- Many supermarkets offer a good selection of frozen (in addition to fresh) organic produce that you can cook and store in large zip-seal bags in the refrigerator and portion them out with each meal.
- Cut up meats, divide them into individual portions, and freeze them in plastic sandwich bags to defrost as needed.

Adding a quality supplement is always a good idea. I designed Canine Everyday Essentials and Vital Vities for Cats for Deserving Pets as completely balanced vitamin, mineral, and superfood supplements. It's microencapsulated so that the ingredients don't oxidize and decay. All you have to do is add the supplement to one of your dog's daily meals.

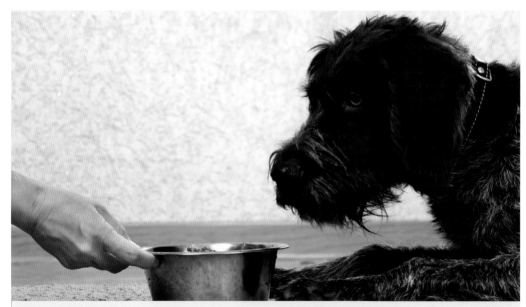

Protein, grains, produce, and a supplement are the components of a healthy diet.

Meal Suggestions and Recipes
Throw-Together Meals

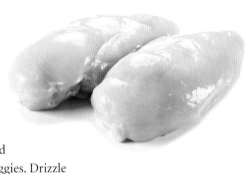

Using the following lists, choose ingredients from each category: proteins, carbohydrates, and vegetables/fruits. Prepare and store them separately. When it's time to fill your dog's beloved food bowl, mix the ingredients together in proportions of one-third protein, one-third carbohydrate, and one-third fruit/veggies. Drizzle the portion with some olive oil or coconut oil, add a supplement, and serve.

Pick a protein: When picking proteins, you're looking for novel proteins (protein sources that your dog has not eaten before). Ideally, you want three novel proteins that you can rotate.

- Rabbit (can buy canned)
- Pork
- Venison
- Bison
- Fish (can buy certain types, such as salmon, canned)
- Turkey
- Lamb
- Goat
- Duck
- Buffalo
- Goat yogurt or goat cheese

Pick a carbohydrate:

- Millet
- Barley
- Brown rice
- Basmati rice
- Sweet potato
- White potato
- Quinoa

Pick one or more vegetables/fruits:

Fruits can include apples, berries (except strawberries), bananas, cantaloupe, and watermelon. Your vegetable choices are endless. Note that the cruciferous vegetables, such as cauliflower, broccoli, brussels sprouts, cabbage, and kale, are anticancer veggies.

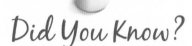

Did You Know?

Goat milk, goat yogurt, and kefir are great choices for snacks or toppings.

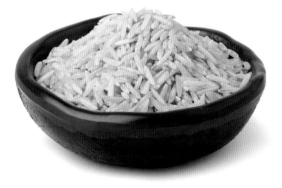

Hypoallergenic Antiyeast Meal

3 cups potatoes, diced
1 cup beef, chicken, lamb, or fish (tilapia or another
   bland white fish), diced
1 cup mixed vegetables (cauliflower, string beans,
   broccoli)
2 cloves garlic
1 tablespoon apple cider vinegar
1/3 cup olive oil

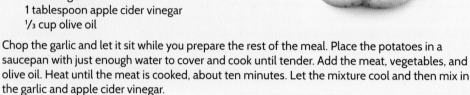

Chop the garlic and let it sit while you prepare the rest of the meal. Place the potatoes in a saucepan with just enough water to cover and cook until tender. Add the meat, vegetables, and olive oil. Heat until the meat is cooked, about ten minutes. Let the mixture cool and then mix in the garlic and apple cider vinegar.

Pork and Beets

1 cup cooked red beet, carrot, or other vegetable,
   chopped
2 sweet potatoes
3/4 cups uncooked brown rice
3 pounds pork cutlets, diced

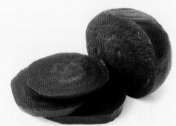

Preheat the oven to 450° F. Coat a large baking dish with olive oil. Put the sweet potatoes in the baking dish, cook in the oven until done, and then mash them. Cook the brown rice until soft, about 45 minutes. Saute the pork cubes in olive oil until they are cooked through. Mix all of the ingredients together and serve.

Rabbit Meat Loaf

1 pound canned or frozen rabbit meat
1/2 cup coconut milk
2 eggs
3/4 cup brown rice flour or cooked brown rice
1 cup frozen organic carrots and peas
1 tablespoon Italian spices

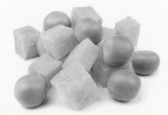

Preheat the oven to 350° F. Beat the eggs and coconut milk together. Mix in the seasonings and rice or flour. Fold in the meat and the frozen vegetables. Bake for 20–25 minutes.

Tuna and Potatoes

1½ pounds tuna
2 cups red potatoes with skin on, diced
½ cup canned pure pumpkin

In a large pot, cover the tuna with water and set the pot over medium heat. Cook for about 20 minutes, until the tuna is cooked through. At the same time, bring a pot of water to boil, add the potatoes, and cook for 20 minutes or until soft. Let all cool. Cut the tuna into small cubes and mix with potatoes. Add the pumpkin, mix all ingredients together, and serve.

White Fish, Oat, and Blueberry Meal in a Muffin

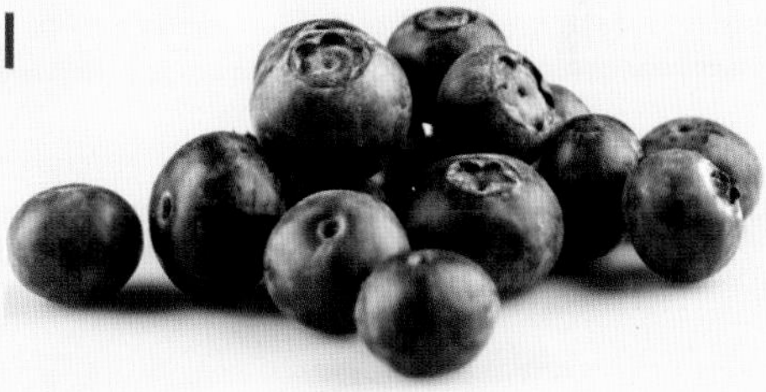

1½ cups coconut flour
6 tablespoons honey
1 tablespoon baking powder
1½ cups rolled oats
1 cup fresh or frozen blueberries
1½ cups fresh or frozen tilapia, cooked and coarsely chopped or flaked
1 cup coconut milk
1 large egg
1 tablespoon olive oil

Preheat the oven to 400° F. Mix the coconut flour and baking powder together, add the oats, and mix. Mix the coconut milk and egg, lightly beating the egg, and add in the honey. Combine these dry and wet ingredients and then fold in the tilapia and blueberries. Bake for 12–15 minutes.

Allergy-Free Muffins

1 cup rice flour
1 teaspoon baking soda
½ cup oat bran
1 cup millet flour
1 cup goat milk
½ cup water

Preheat oven to 400° F. Mix the dry ingredients together. Mix the wet ingredients in a separate bowl. Combine the wet and dry ingredients and then spoon the batter into oiled muffin tins. Bake for 40 minutes.

Oatmeal Breakfast

1 cup cooked oatmeal
¼ cup fresh or frozen blueberries
1 tablespoon honey
¼ cup goat milk or goat yogurt

Mix blueberries, honey, and goat milk/yogurt into cooked oatmeal and serve.

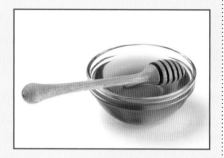

Potatoes au Canine

3 cups potatoes, boiled and sliced
¼ cup cheese of your choice, grated
½ cup cottage cheese
2 tablespoons vegetables of your choice, grated
¼ cup whole milk

Preheat oven to 350°F. Place a layer of potato slices at the bottom of a buttered square casserole dish. Spread half of the cottage cheese over the layer of potatoes and then add another layer of potatoes. Spread the rest of the cottage cheese over the top layer of potatoes. Pour the milk over the layered mixture and top with grated cheese and grated vegetables. Bake until the cheese is melted and slightly browned, which usually takes 15–20 minutes.

Tarragon Fish Hearty Man Stew (Grain-Free and Gluten-Free)

1 large white fish, frozen or fresh
¼ cup olive oil
3 cups carrots, sliced
3 cups potatoes, cubed
4 parsnips, sliced
2 cups broccoli stems, sliced
6 cloves garlic, sliced
1 teaspoon tarragon

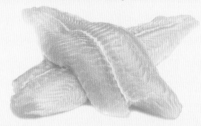

Place white fish in a large pot with 2 quarts of water, bring to a boil, and then reduce to a simmer and cook until the meat is tender. Cool the white fish, remove the meat from the bones, and return the meat to the pot. Add the olive oil, carrots, potatoes, parsnips, garlic, tarragon, and broccoli stems. Return to a boil and then simmer again for 30 minutes. Remove from heat, cool, and serve. Divide the rest into meal-sized portions in zipper-sealed bags and refrigerate or freeze.

Fruits of the Sea Hearty Man Stew (Gluten-Free)

2 pounds tilapia, cubed
1 flat sheet kombu seaweed
3 tablespoons parsley
5 cloves garlic, sliced
2 cups carrots, sliced
4 cups basmati or jasmine white rice (replace with 4 cups cubed white potatoes for grain-free)

Fill a stockpot with 3 quarts of water. Add all ingredients to the pot, bring to a boil, and then simmer for 30 minutes. Cool, remove sheet of kombu, and serve. Divide the rest into meal-sized portions in zipper-sealed bags and refrigerate or freeze.

Sweet Potatoes and Rabbit (Grain-Free and Gluten-Free)

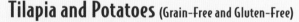

4 sweet potatoes, skinned
3 cups boneless rabbit
1 cup grated vegetable of your choice

Preheat oven to 400°F and bake the skinned sweet potatoes for 60–90 minutes or until thoroughly cooked. Cut the rabbit into pieces and cook however you like (except frying). Mash the cooked sweet potatoes and mix in the cooked rabbit pieces and grated vegetables. Serve when cool. Refrigerate leftovers, covered, for up to three days.

Tilapia and Potatoes (Grain-Free and Gluten-Free)

1 pound fresh tilapia or other white fish
4 cups white potatoes; skin on, chopped
1 teaspoon dried rosemary
1/3 cup olive oil

Place the potatoes in a large pot with the rosemary, olive oil, and enough unsalted water to just cover the potatoes. Bring to boil and cook until the potatoes are tender. Slice the fish into strips and add it to the potatoes and water. Mix in well and bring to a boil again for another 10–15 minutes or until the fish is cooked through. Remove from heat, cool, and serve.

Salmon and Potatoes (Grain-Free and Gluten-Free)

3 medium potatoes
1 can low-salt salmon
1/2 cup grated carrot

Cook potatoes however you desire. Add in the salmon and carrots and mix well. Serve when cool. Refrigerate leftovers, covered, for up to three days.

Quinoa, Cauliflower, and Tasty Turkey

1 cup quinoa
turkey parts (thighs and/or wings)
1 cup cauliflower, chopped
2 tablespoons fresh parsley, chopped
⅓ cup olive oil

Rinse the quinoa with tap water to remove any bitter taste from the outside husks and set aside. Place 4 cups of water in a saucepan and add the turkey pieces. Bring to a boil and then simmer, covered, until the turkey is cooked. Cool. Remove the turkey bones and place the turkey meat back into the water. Add the quinoa, cauliflower pieces, and olive oil. Bring back to a boil and immediately reduce to a simmer, covered, for 30 minutes. Remove from heat and mix in the parsley. Let cool and serve.

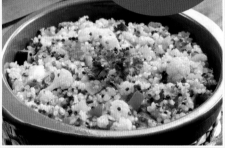

Quinoa is a grain with high protein content. It is also a complete protein. This grain was historically grown in the Andes Mountains of South America.

Mackerel and Oatmeal

3 cups steel-cut oats, cooked
12–16-ounce can mackerel
3 tablespoons fresh parsley, chopped, or 2 teaspoons of dried parsley

Place 1 cup of the steel-cut oats in 3½ cups of water. Bring to a quick boil and then simmer on very low heat for 30–40 minutes, checking regularly and adding more water if needed. Put oatmeal in a large bowl, fluff it up, and allow it to cool a bit. Add the canned mackerel, parsley, and rest of oatmeal and mix. Finish cooling and serve.

Venison and Potatoes (Grain-Free and Gluten-Free)

3 cups potatoes, skin on, diced
1 cup venison, cubed
1 cup frozen peas and carrots
⅓ cup olive oil
½ teaspoon powdered rosemary

Place the diced potatoes in a large pot and fill with just enough unsalted water to cover the potatoes. Bring to a boil and then simmer until the potatoes are soft. Add the cubed venison, rosemary, and olive oil and simmer for another 10 minutes. Add the frozen peas and carrots and simmer for another 10 minutes. Remove from heat, cool, and serve.

Feeding Your Allergic Cat

Our finicky felines do very well with raw meat. That said, cats with chronic GI symptoms might be more susceptible to pathogens in the meat. The prevailing thought used to be that freezing killed these pathogens, but a group of researchers from the Netherlands checked samples from thirty-five raw-meat pet products from eight different brands and found that 23 percent of these products were contaminated with a type of *E. coli* that can cause renal failure in humans. This study, published in the January 2018 issue of the British Veterinary Association's *Veterinary Record*, also found that 80 percent of products contained antibiotic-resistant strains of *E. coli* and that varying percentages of the products contained *Listeria*, *Salmonella*, and other dangerous pathogens. Many of the pet-food companies tested sold frozen raw meat, which means that freezing did not kill the bugs in the meat and poultry. That's why raw meat may be pushing the envelope as a diet for cats who already have gastrointestinal problems.

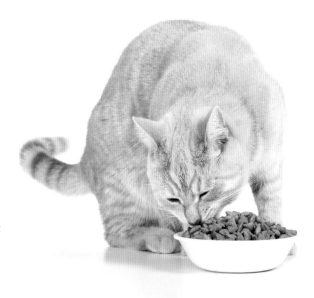

We know that fish is commonly used as an ingredient to flavor cat foods, but many cats are allergic to fish. Even if the cat-food label lists chicken or lamb as the main ingredient, you will likely also find some type of fish or salmon oil in the ingredient list.

To add insult to injury, the type of fish commonly used in cat foods is tilefish, often euphemistically listed on labels as "ocean whitefish." The manufacturers do this because tilefish is one of the worst, along with tuna, king mackerel, shark, and swordfish, as far as containing toxic levels of mercury. The United States Environmental Protection Agency and Food and Drug Administration both release advisories about consuming certain types of fish due to health concerns about mercury, proving that the risk is very real. Both organizations advise limiting fish intake and choosing fish species that are lower in mercury.

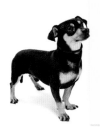

Did You Know?

Organ meats from a species will often not create problem for pets who are sensitive or intolerant to that species; for example, a pet who is sensitive to chicken will likely be able to eat chicken liver.

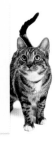

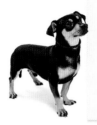

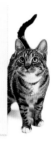

Did You Know?

If you are making a transition from wet food or kibble, you can begin by reducing the amount of commercial food and adding proportionally more meat and then the the other ingredients until the food is completely switched over.

The pet-food company Farmina sells a hypoallergenic cat food called UltraHypo that required a prescription from your vet. Other companies offer prepared hypoallergenic meals made for cats. For example, an online company called Smalls makes a meal for cats with turkey breast, chicken livers, peas, kale, and spinach. There are other companies that create organic, healthy cat meals; you just have to choose your ingredients carefully.

Designing the Feline Diet

Pick a Protein: The same principle applies to cats as to dogs. You want to choose a novel protein (one that your cat has not eaten before). Ideally, you can find three novel proteins that you can rotate.

By far, my favorite protein for cats with itching or chronic GI problems is rabbit. It has only one phenolic in it and does not contain the notorious gallic acid. You can buy rabbit-based commercial foods for cats as well as canned rabbit. If you choose a commercial kibble, you'll need to read the label carefully to check for any added ingredients that can cause problems.

Choose a protein/proteins from the following:

- Rabbit
- Pork
- Venison
- Bison
- Fish (mild whitefish or salmon), if your cat does not already have an intolerance to fish
- Turkey
- Duck
- Lamb
- Goat
- Buffalo
- Goat yogurt or goat cheese

You don't have too many choices for carbohydrates and vegetables for cats because we're limiting ingredients and because cats can be really picky. That doesn't mean that you can't try out some starches and vegetables that are not listed in the following recipes.

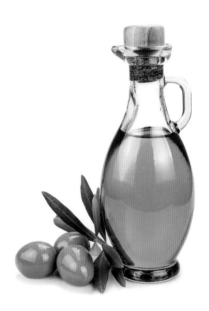

Simple Recipe for Cats

Protein: 3 ounces cooked rabbit, pork, lamb, or duck
Carbohydrate: ⅓ cup cooked white rice or peas (such as organic baby-food peas)
Fiber: ⅕ cup cooked sweet potato, without skin, or summer squash (such as organic baby-food squash is great)
Fat (optional): ¼ teaspoon olive oil
Supplement: Vital Vities for Cats by Deserving Pets

Mix all ingredients together and serve.

Delicious Duck

4½ pounds cooked whole duck
6 jars organic baby-food carrots

Bake the duck in the oven at 350° F until tender. Let cool and then remove the bones and skin. Dice the cooled duck into very small pieces and then coat the duck with the carrots. Divide into individual portions and store. Before serving, sprinkle Vital Vities supplement on the food.

Turkey and Pumpkin

6 pounds cooked boneless dark-meat turkey, finely chopped
2 cups pumpkin puree
2 tablespoons olive oil
8 ounces of cooked, finely chopped chicken liver—can cook by lightly sautéing in olive oil

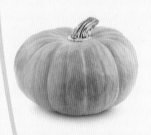

Mix turkey and chicken liver together and let cool if necessary. Mix in the pumpkin puree. Divide into individual portions and store. Before serving, sprinkle Vital Vities supplement on the food.

Gelatin Treat for Cats

½ cup unflavored gelatin (**Important:** Only use *unflavored* gelatin.)
½ cup cold water
1½ cups broth of your choice (e.g., rabbit, turkey, fish)

Add the gelatin to the cold water let it stand to soften. Bring the broth to a boil and pour over the gelatin; stir until gelatin dissolves. Pour the mixture into a 9- x 12-inch pan and let it harden. Cut it into tiny bite-sized pieces and give them to your cat as treats.

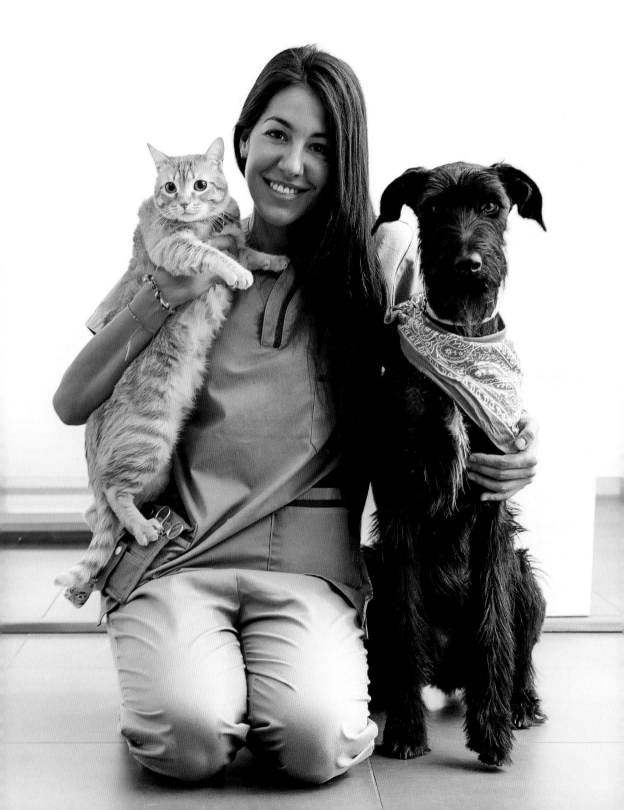

Appendix I

Core and Noncore Dog and Cat Vaccinations Recommended by Dr. Jean Dodds

Core Vaccination Protocol for Dogs

9–10 weeks of age:
- Distemper and parvovirus MLV (modified live-virus)

14 weeks of age:
- Distemper and parvovirus MLV

18 weeks of age:
- Single monovalent parvovirus only

20 weeks of age or older, if allowable by law:
- Rabies

1 year of age:
- Distemper and parvovirus MLV booster (or optional titer)

1 year after initial rabies vaccination:
- Rabies, killed three-year booster (thimerosol-free), given three to four weeks apart from distemper/parvovirus booster

Every three years thereafter (or more often, if desired), have titers for distemper and parvovirus performed. Vaccinate for rabies according to the law. If the law allows you to obtain a rabies exemption waiver from your veterinarian, have a rabies titer test performed at the time of requesting the waiver.

Core Vaccination Protocol for Cats

8–9 weeks of age:
- FVRCP

12–13 weeks of age:
- FVRCP

24 weeks of age or older, if required by law:
- Rabies

1 year of age:
- FVRCP booster

1 year after initial rabies vaccination:
- Rabies, two to three weeks apart from FVRCP

Every three years thereafter (or more often, if desired), have titers for panleukopenia virus performed. Vaccinate for rabies according to the law. If the law allows you to obtain a rabies exemption waiver from your veterinarian, have a rabies titer test performed at the time of requesting the waiver.

Noncore Vaccines for Dogs
Lyme Disease

I do not recommend the Lyme vaccine. I have had many patients who have been vaccinated for Lyme disease on the appropriate schedule and who have then contracted the disease. One reason for this is that Lyme disease is caused by bacteria, and vaccines for bacterial diseases don't provide extended coverage. In truth, you need to vaccinate up to four times a year to truly provide protection. Vaccinating on that kind of schedule becomes both prohibitive and dangerous.

The first thing to know is that 85 to 95 percent of dogs infected with Lyme bacteria by a tick do not get Lyme disease. The second thing to understand is that Lyme disease can, in both humans and dogs, cause autoimmune problems, and the vaccine actually increases this risk. One common problem in dogs with Lyme disease is a kidney disease called *Lyme nephritis* or *autoimmune glomerulonephritis*. This kidney disease is an immune-mediated response to the infectious agents, or antigens, introduced to the body via either Lyme disease or the Lyme vaccine. The dog's immune system attacks its own kidney tubules and eats away little holes, called *glomeruli*, in these tubules.

Research from Cornell University Veterinary School cites the long-term side effects from Lyme vaccination, which can include rheumatoid arthritis, any or all of the symptoms of Lyme disease itself, and potential death due to kidney failure. Side effects usually occur within four to eight weeks of vaccination.

Authorities on veterinary vaccines do not recommend the Lyme disease vaccine; instead, they emphasize the importance of keeping your dog free of ticks. Remember, unlike a virus such as distemper, in which a correctly timed vaccination schedule will provide lifetime immunity, the Lyme vaccine is vaccinating against a bacteria; therefore, the protection is negligible and short-lived. Once again, you'd have to vaccinate at least twice a year with a vaccine that in itself poses many dangers. Because the number of dogs who actually contract Lyme disease is very low, I feel that the Lyme vaccine is an unnecessary health risk.

Natural Tick Repellent

A produce by PetzLife called Herbal Defense comes in a topical coat spray as well as in a powder that is added to your pet's food. The herbal formula is completely natural and nontoxic, and it is effective in keeping fleas, ticks, and other external parasites off dogs and cats.

Leptospirosis

Leptospirosis is an uncommon disease which, when diagnosed, is easily treated. Again, unlike viral vaccines, which likely last for the life of the animal, bacterial vaccines such as "lepto" persist for less than a year, so many veterinarians recommend vaccinating every six months. Leading veterinary

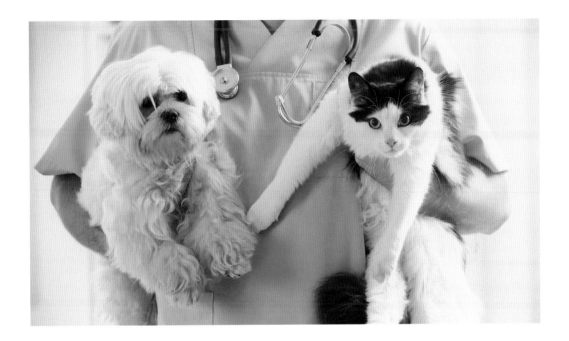

immunologist Ronald D. Schultz, PhD, said that you might even need to give this vaccine as often as four times a year.

The problem is that the lepto vaccine involves a high level of risk for your dog. I used to order routine combination vaccinations without the leptospirosis components because the lepto vaccine was making dogs sick after vaccination. In fact, many veterinarians, conventional and holistic alike, avoided the leptospirosis part of vaccines because they didn't want to risk the complications that occur so commonly after vaccinating for lepto.

Additionally, there's actually a chance that your dog won't be protected by the vaccine because there are twenty different species of *Leptospira* bacteria and more than two hundred different serovars. The current vaccines contain *L. canicola*, *L. icterohaemorrhagiae*, *L. grippotyphosa*, and *L. pomona*. Two additional serovars that appear to cause infection, *L. bratislava* and *L. automalis*, are not included in the vaccines currently available. So if you do decide to vaccinate your dog, it's a

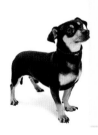

Did You Know?

About 30 percent of dogs do not respond to the lepto vaccine with immunity. It's important to know that dogs can actually get the disease from vaccination, and they can then shed the virus and spread the disease to other dogs.

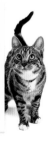

very good idea to find out which strains of leptospirosis are in your area so that you don't give your dog a risky vaccination that won't even protect him.

The side effects of the vaccine, in my opinion, far outweigh any potential benefit. Proven complications from the leptospirosis vaccination include lameness, fever, polyarthritis, kidney failure, liver failure, pancreatitis, mast cell disease, urinary tract infections, enlarged spleen, enlarged lymph nodes, diarrhea, chronic weight loss, cancer, and even death.

Bordetella (Kennel Cough)

Once again, I refer to the renowned veterinary immunologist, Dr. Ronald Schultz. In an article on the *Dogs Naturally Magazine* blog, Dana Scott quotes Dr. Schultz as saying, "Kennel cough is not a vaccinatable disease."

The kennel cough vaccine is, in fact, relatively ineffective. The intranasal form works better than the injection, but it still isn't very effective. The vaccine cannot offer protection against the disease; it only lessens the severity of the upper respiratory infection caused by *Bordetella*. And if it did actually work, it would be effective for only up to three months at a time, necessitating vaccination four times a year. *Bordetella* is a bacteria, not a virus.

Vaccinated dogs can still shed the upper respiratory bug into the environment, infecting other unsuspecting pups. Plus, the intranasal vaccine has been known to cause complications, such as collapsing trachea and pneumonia.

If your dog doesn't go to kennels, doggy daycare, or groomers, he is very unlikely to contract kennel cough. Additionally, it's a self-limiting disease, sort of like a cold. Lastly, it's very easy to treat kennel cough. Your dog will exhibit only minor symptoms and will be fine after five to seven days if you give him one of the following homeopathic remedies:

- Antimonium tart 6x or 30x, four times a day
- Drosera 6x or 30x, four to six times a day
- Belladonna 6x, three to four times a day (recommended for dogs with low-grade fevers)
- Colloidal silver, three tablespoons, three times a day

Colloidal Silver

Colloidal silver can have miraculous results with many types of infections. I recommend Argentyn 23®, a professional-grade formula.

Canine Influenza

Veterinary clinics and the news have made the canine flu very scary. Let's start with the history. The initial virus, H3N8, started in horses and transmuted to infect dogs at a Greyhound track. From there, it rapidly spread to forty states. Some cats in an Indiana shelter actually came down with the virus, too. Then, H3N2, which was originally a bird virus starting in Asia, caused a dog flu outbreak in Chicago in 2015.

The press makes it sound sort of dire. During the Chicago-area outbreak, there were supposedly five deaths out of more than one thousand cases reported. But it turned out that two of the five dogs had died from the canine flu vaccine rather than from the flu itself.

According to Julia Henriques on the *Dogs Naturally* blog, Dr. Jean Dodds believes the real fatality rate is 2 to 3 percent while maintaining that only dogs who are compromised in some way (such as by malnutrition, parasites, or other health problems) are at risk of dying from the flu. Healthy animals are expected to recover completely in about two weeks.

Even I would be wondering, *Well, if my dog can die from this, maybe I should vaccinate…* So let's discuss the protection that the vaccine affords your dog. Remember, there are two different canine flu viruses: the original H3N8 and the newer H3N2. The original canine flu vaccine contained only the H3N8 virus. At the end of 2015, pharmaceutical companies rushed the H3N2 vaccine to market with conditional licenses from the USDA, meaning that studies were still in progress to determine the efficacy and safety of the vaccine.

Additionally, flu viruses mutate year after year. That's why there's a new flu vaccine every year for humans. The previous year's vaccination wouldn't work because the disease-causing virus changes rapidly. Human flu vaccines have an effectiveness rate of only about 50 percent even though they are updated every year. The canine flu vaccine is not updated regularly, so its efficacy rate is likely lower.

Just as with kennel cough, there are effective treatments that nip the flu in the bud and shorten the duration of the illness dramatically. The homeopathic remedy Phosphorus 30c, given four times a day, is proven to reduce the duration and severity of the flu to as little as a week of mild symptoms.

It's important to look at your pet's lifestyle when deciding whether to vaccinate. Flu usually occurs where dogs live or spend time closely together, such as boarding kennels, shelters, and doggy daycare. If your dog is not at risk, I would advise against this vaccine. If your dog will be in a risky situation, such as at a dog show, I would advise giving him a form of lauric acid called monolaurin, which offers protection against viral infections. Give monolaurin twice a day for one day before and during the time of potential exposure.

Noncore Vaccines for Cats
Feline Leukemia Virus (FeLV) Vaccine

FeLV is *not* highly contagious, and its transmission requires prolonged and intimate contact with an infected cat. Natural immunity, without ever having had a vaccination, is very strong in most cats by the age of one year. Conventional guidelines recommend vaccinating all kittens, but vaccinating an adult cat is recommended only if she will be in contact with a known FeLV-positive cat.

FeLV is considered a noncore vaccination. Dr. Ronald Schultz recommends this vaccination for cats at risk, and his reasoning is very sound. Dr. Schultz recommends FeLV vaccination initially at ten weeks and then again at fourteen weeks. After that, you never need to vaccinate again. He feels that just these two doses would make a tremendous difference in the occurrence of FeLV in cats—if enough kittens were vaccinated at ten and fourteen weeks, we could effectively eradicate the disease.

Also trust that two vaccinations are totally enough for complete protection. If one persists in giving vaccines the incidence of Vaccine Associated Sarcoma will increase.

Important!

Never mix vaccinations. Give only one combination shot, such as the FVRCP, and do not combine it with rabies or any noncore vaccination. It may take more veterinary visits, but it is much safer for your cat.

Feline Infectious Peritonitis (FIP) Vaccine

FIP is a complex disease caused by a coronavirus. Research shows that just about every cat has this virus in her system, but it becomes pathogenic in some cats, causing the fatal symptoms of FIP. Research also shows that the thymus gland, an important part of the immune system, becomes ineffectual and incapable before FIP occurs.

In my opinion, the vaccine is not effective and is dangerous to give. Very few veterinarians recommend or give this vaccination.

Feline Immunodeficiency Virus (FIV or Feline AIDS)

This is a very ineffective vaccination and is not likely to provide immunity to the disease. Plus, a vaccinated cat will test positive for the disease because the test cannot tell the difference between the disease and the vaccination. Therefore, if your cat becomes sick and tests positive for FIV, you won't know for sure if FIV is really the problem. Very few veterinarians recommend or give this vaccine. I do not recommend it.

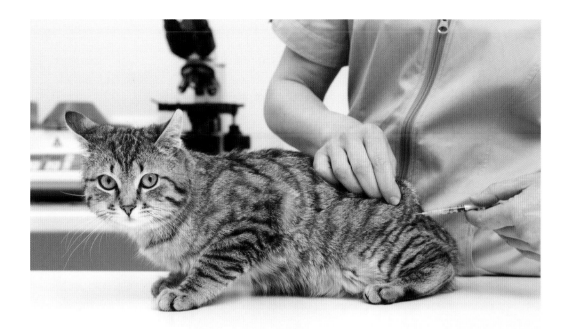

Chlamydiosis

Chlamydiosis is caused by the bacteria *Chlamydia psittaci*. This bacteria can cause conjunctivitis along with sneezing and nasal discharge. It is transmitted through direct contact with an infected cat. The same situation exists in which cats have high natural immunity to this disease by one year of age. Similar to the canine kennel cough vaccine, the chlamydiosis vaccine does not prevent infection; rather, it lessens the severity of the symptoms. Importantly, adverse reactions associated with this vaccination are more prevalent than with many of the other feline vaccines.

Other Vaccines

Vaccinations are available for *Bordetella* and *Giardia*, but neither is widely recommended. Both conditions are uncommon in pet cats, and both respond well to treatment. Further, the *Giardia* vaccine is associated with vaccine-site reactions due to added components in the vaccine.

Rabies

Rabies needs to be boosted one year after the first vaccine and then every three years. If you have a cat who lives solely indoors, you can discuss the need for the rabies vaccine with your veterinarian.

Appendix II

A Guide to Administering Homeopathic Remedies

Doses of homeopathic remedies are not adjusted for size or weight as, let's say, an antibiotic or herbal remedy would be. In homeopathy, the potency, or number of times the remedy was diluted, and the frequency of the doses are what matter. In most cases, as soon as the symptoms improve, the remedy has done its job and can be discontinued.

Because the original physical substance is sequentially diluted, there is a number after the name of the remedy. For example, Arnica 6x does not mean that you have to give it six times. It means that the remedy has been diluted six times, and the "x" stands for a dilution ratio of 1:10. If you see a "c" after the remedy's name, it indicates a dilution ratio of 1:100. Further, the more dilute the remedy, the more powerful it is, so very highly diluted remedies are usually available only to doctors. The potencies most commonly available to consumers are 6x and 30x (diluted 1:10 either six or thirty times) and 6c and 30c (diluted 1:100 either six or thirty times).

Everything that touches a homeopathic remedy should be clean and odor free. You may hear that you cannot handle the remedies, but this is not true. As long as your hands are clean, you can handle the remedies without a problem. I have been doing this for more than thirty years with no problems.

Homeopathic remedies are available as either a water-based liquid, which is often preserved with a little alcohol or vinegar, or as small white tablets or pellets that are coated with the remedy. Both dogs and cats usually do not mind the taste of these preparations, although they may resist the

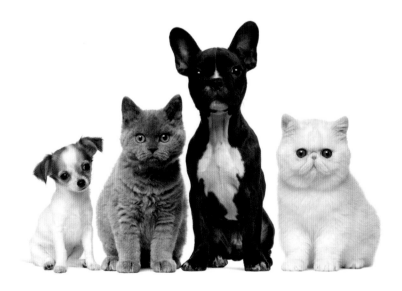

Storage Tips

- If you spill the remedy, avoid contamination by discarding the spilled portion. Do not put it back into the bottle.
- Keep pellets at room temperature. You can refrigerate homemade liquid preparations.
- Keep homeopathic remedies away from computers and microwaves

higher-alcohol liquid preparations, which you can dilute with water before administering if needed. Remedies need to melt on the mucous membranes of the mouth, either on the gums or inside the lips, and therefore should not be hidden in the pet's food. If using a liquid preparation, you drop the liquid under your pet's lip, onto the gums. Place some of the remedy into a 1- or 2-ounce dropper bottle (preferably amber) with some water, and use the dropper to administer the remedy. If using the tablets/pellets, you can easily insert them into your pet's lip fold to allow them to dissolve and absorb—this is much easier than having to pry your pet's mouth open to push a pill down his or her throat.

The size of the tablets and pellets vary. In my practice, I use the very tiny #15 size pellets, which are so small that they stick to a cat's or dog's gums so that the pet can't spit them out. Dogs often spit out larger tablets and pellets, and the larger sizes do not work at all with cats. You can do one of two things with the larger pellets: (1) crush them in a small folded piece of paper and then use the folded paper to slide the powder into the pet's mouth, or (2) add several pellets to a 1- or 2-ounce dropper bottle with some water and shake to make a liquid preparation of the remedy just as in above. Make a new, fresh liquid preparation about every week because they contain no preservatives.

Do not give homeopathic remedies at mealtimes, and never mix them into your pet's food. Ideally, you should administer the remedy at least twenty minutes before or twenty minutes after your pet eats. If your schedule allows you to wait only five minutes, it is OK, but twenty minutes or more is optimal.

Follow your practitioner's instructions on how often to give the remedy. The most important thing to remember is that the number of pills/tablets or drops of liquid is not critical. You can give one tablet to an elephant and ten to a mouse. The size of the pills is also not important. You are administering the *energy* of the medicine and not the actual *material substance* of that medicine. It is more important to select the right remedy than to worry about precise dosing.

Appendix III

Allergy Elimination 4 Pets Procedure

The common practice is for me to consult with the pet owners and prepare a program of vials that is specifically tailored to each pet. If you wish to do the treatment without a consult, you can use preprepared vials that cover most of what I commonly find in our pets. Available at Deserving Pets (*www.deservingpets.com*), they contain energetic resonances of the most common things to which our pets are allergic.

You don't have to face a lifetime of food avoidance, special baths, and all the other things that are part and parcel of caring for an allergic dog or cat. It's time to turn your pet into a nonallergic pet. It may sound too good to be true, but my Allergy Elimination 4 Pets technique is a remarkably effective holistic modality to treat allergies.

Here are the ingredients in the vials I have prepared for you:

1. Vaccines Dog (or Vaccines Cat)
2. Chicken/Egg/Turkey/Duck
3. Calcium/Dairy Mix/Cheese Mix
4. B Vitamins/Yeast Mix/Grains
5. All Grains/Wheat/Gluten
6. Meat Mix: Lamb, Beef, Pork, Veal, Venison
7. Fish and Shellfish Mix
8. Corn and Soy
9. Mold and Fungus Mix
10. Grass Mix
11. Tree Mix/Pollen Mix
12. Weed Mix
13. Dust/Dust Mites
14. Potato Rice

Author's note: There is a vial (Vial D) for chronic diarrhea that is included for pets with GI problems.

In my practice, I test each pet to find the exact items to which they are reacting, and I treat them. I then check if the previous treatment was successful and move on to the next item. In treating your pet, as far as the items I've prepared for you, I am going to ask you to treat each item several times to ensure that the treatment is complete.

You don't have to do the treatments according to the numbers on the vials. If it's obvious to you that your pet is allergic to grains or chicken, you can start with that item. In some cases, you may be treating for an item to which your pet isn't allergic, but it will do no harm at all. I'm simply trying to cover all of the bases for most pets.

You will treat each item once a day for three days at bedtime or sometime before bedtime because we want to avoid the problem food (as best we can) for forty-eight hours after treating for it. Treating at bedtime or right after dinner gives you twelve to sixteen hours of avoidance overnight (or longer if you feed your pet only once per day), and this time often is sufficient to allow your

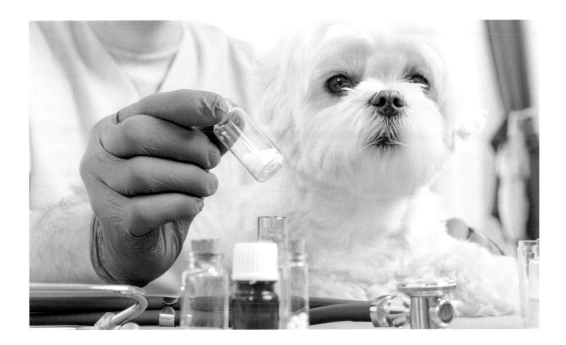

pet's system to readjust and correct its reaction to the allergen. If you leave food out for your pet, take it away. Play it safe.

If, when you are done with the treatment, you find that your pet is much better but not 100 percent cured, you can treat him or her with items from your own home. Here are some examples:

1. Take a tablespoon of vacuum-cleaner dirt right from the vacuum bag and place it in a small, clean glass jar. Use it like one of the vials and treat accordingly.
2. Place a wide-mouthed plastic container, such as a deli container, outside with ½ inch (1¼ cm)or so of water in it and leave it for twenty-four to forty-eight hours. The water will gather pollen. Put the water in a small glass jar and treat, using it as you would one of the vials.
3. Do the same as #2 but leave the container indoors.

While the Grass, Pollen, Tree, and Weed Mixes are quite complete, they can't cover every plant on the planet. If your pet's allergies are exacerbated at a certain time of year, do #2 at that time of year. You can also gather plants in your area or on your property that you think might be culprits, make a small bouquet, and treat.

Note: If your pet is itchy in the spring and fall, it's likely that food allergies are lurking below that threshold line. If you treat just the seasonal environmental items, the treatment may not work very well.

Importantly, if you find that your pet is not improving or is not 100 percent cured, you can (1) go through the protocol once more, (2) make sure that there is not an "allergy copycat" such as malassezia, at work, (3) contact me for a professional consult so that I can review your pet's case (there is a consultation fee), or (4) try doing the B vitamins for one week, treating once a night for seven nights. If your pet has chronic diarrhea, you treat with Vial D once a day for one week. If itchiness and/or diarrhea still persist, there is no substitute for a thorough veterinary exam with your local veterinarian.

Treatment Notes

1. Keep the vials away from electronic devices, such as computers and microwaves. The vials will be good to use for one year after receipt.
2. The vials are usually, but not always, done in order. If you do them out of order, keep notes or a calendar.
3. It may be difficult to avoid having your pet eat or contact the specific allergens for which they are being treated for the twenty-four hours after the treatment. Sometimes, such as in the case of pollen, dust, or mold, it is just impossible; it is easier when treating for food items. B vitamins are one of the most difficult items to both avoid and cure.
4. Treat each vial for three days in a row and then move to the next vial.
5. You can take a break whenever you need to. For example, you can decide to treat one allergen for three days each week, taking four days off each week. It will just take a bit longer to complete the entire treatment.

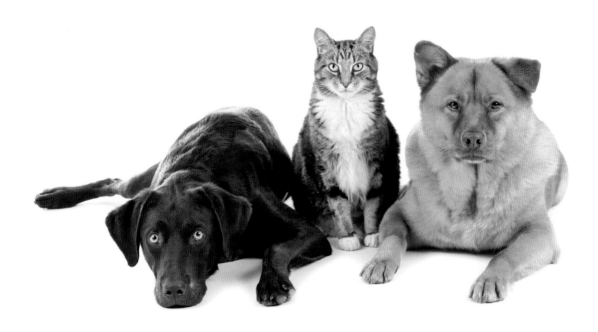

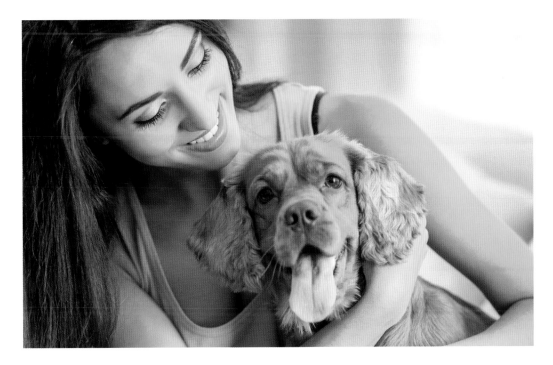

Treatment Procedure

1. The glass part of the vial needs to be next to your dog or cat. You can accomplish this by placing the vial snugly under the collar if your pet wears one; we have included a tiny bag that you can put the vial in and attach to the collar. Alternately, you can sit your pet on your lap and place or hold the vial next to him or her. The best way is to hold it with your flat hand right against your pet's belly. If your pet is lying down, you can just tuck it under his belly.

2. Create a "U" shape with your thumb and forefinger.

3. Starting just below the neck (above the shoulder), tap by applying light, gentle, but recognizable pressure with the thumb and forefinger on either side of the spine. Now move down about 1 inch and tap again. The pressure is about the same as pressing a key on your computer's keyboard. (**Note:** If your cat is reactive, tap very, very gently.) Continue to repeat until you reach the top of the tail. Two long strips of muscles sit immediately on either side of the vertebral column, so you are tapping gently on these muscles, which are acupuncture points. It should be a massaging, rather than a "knocking," action. (You will receive an instructional video along with your vials.)

4. Repeat the process of tapping from top to bottom, with the vial next to your pet, twenty times.

5. After you finish tapping, keep the vial next to your pet for five or more minutes. This should be a quiet and peaceful time.

6. Remove the vial and place it back in the kit.

7. Repeat these steps each evening for three evenings per vial.

Index

fish oil, 168

fish-based food, 133

flea prevention, 65–71

    evaluation of situation, 67–68

    general discussion, 65–66

    natural alternatives, 68–69

    risks, 70–71, 108

    spot-on products, 67–70

food allergies

    delayed responses, 41

    food sensitivities and
      intolerances versus, 8, 25–31

    overview, 8

    testing for, 42, 176–177

Food and Drug Administration
  (FDA), 199

foods, 125–137

    carbohydrates, 193

    for cats, 199–201

    commercial, 127, 200

    common, 202

    diets (*See* diets and dietary
      decisions)

    fish-based, 133

    fruits, 193

    glyphosates, 74, 129–131

    harmful to dogs, 191

    meal size, 190–191

    meal suggestions, 193

    meat, 132–134

    organ meats, 199

    phenolics in, 126, 202

    promoting alkaline
      pH in, 116

    proteins, 193

    raw, 10, 134, 199

    variety, 191–192

    vegetables, 193

    wheat, 128–129

See also diets and dietary
  decisions; recipes;
  supplements

Franklin, Benjamin, 63

Fruit of the Sea Hearty Man Stew,
  197

fruits, 193

fungal infections, 94

FVRCP vaccination, 50, 51, 52,
  57, 59

G

GALT (gut-associated lymphoid
  tissue), 119

Gardner, Robert, 27

garlic, 45, 71

garlic acid, 28–29, 31, 156

gastrointestinal problems

    constipation, 151, 160–161

    D3 vitamins and, 152–155

    diarrhea, 98–99, 151,
      155–159

    general discussion, 151–152

    irritable bowel disease, 154

    vomiting, 151, 159–160

Gelatin Treat for Cats, 201

Giardia, 100, 209

glucans, 120

glutathione, 110

gluten intolerance, 128

glyphosates, 74, 129–131

Goodhart, George, 176, 177

Goose's story, 10–12

Graphites, 147

Grindelia, 143, 145

growth hormones, 115

gut. *See* intestines

gut flora, 121

H

heartworm preventives, 67

Hemopet laboratory, 58, 108

Henriques, Julia, 207

Hepar suph, 147

Herbal Defense Spray, 70, 204

herbicides, 74, 129

Higa, Teruo, 42, 45

histamines, 26, 34, 139–140

HistoPlex-AB, 171

holistic health, 18

    approach to drugs, 164

    energetic holistic medicine, 173

    holistic products, 81

    overview, 17–19

    springtime liver cleanse, 118

    thyroid problems and, 108

homeopathic remedies

    administering, 210

    for desensitizing to phenolics, 31

    for diarrhea, 155–156

    for hot spots, 147

    for itching, 145

hookworms, 100, 101

hormones, in food, 132, 134

hot spots, 146–147

Hypoallergenic Antiyeast Meal, 194

hypothyroidism, 107–109

I

IDEXX laboratory, 108

imidacloprid (flea and tick
  treatment), 68

immune system, 21–23, 35, 119,
  181–185

    See also autoimmune diseases;
      Jaffe-Mellor Technique (JMT)

immunoglobulin A, 26, 40–41, 127

immunoglobulin E, 26, 33–34

immunoglobulin G, 26, 33–34

immunoglobulin M, 26, 40–41, 127

indole, 31

influenza, canine, 206–207

inhalant allergies, 37

inoculations. *See* vaccinations

International College of Applied Kinesiology (ICAK), 176

intestines, 39–45
  allergies and, 26
  glucans, 120
  immunoglobulins, 40–41
  importance of, 118–120
  irritable bowel disease, 39–40
  microorganisms, 42–45
  mycoplasmas, 41
  prebiotics, 121
  probiotics, 44, 120–123, 157
  transfer factors, 120

intolerance, to foods, 25–31

Ipecac, 160

irritable bowel disease (IBD), 7, 39, 151–152

itching, causes of, 33-34, 37, 139-140, 146-147

itching, remedies for, 139-149
  allergy rinse or spray, 149
  aloe vera, 142, 147
  baking soda, 141–142
  black tea, 144
  cabbage leaf, 144
  Calendula officinalis, 140–141
  coat refresher, 149
  colloidal oatmeal, 144
  enzyme products, 144
  Grindelia tincture, 143
  homepathic remedies, 145
  Japanese green tea, 144

lavender, 148
  oil-controlling rinse or spray, 149
  PetAlive Allergy Itch Ease, 144
  phenolic remedies, 144
  Preparation H cream, 144
  witch hazel, 142
  zinc oxide ointment, 144

J

Jaffe, Carolyn, 43, 184

Jaffe-Mellor Technique (JMT), 43, 184–185
  See also immune system

JAKs (Janus kinases), 85–86

Japanese green tea, 144

Journal of Clinical Oncology, 134

K

Kaopectate, 155

kennel cough (bordetella), 206, 209

kennel cough vaccine, 56–57

kinases, 85

Kirk's Current Veterinary Therapy I (Schultz & Phillips), 49

kittens, vaccinations, 50–52, 59

kudzu, 157, 159

L

lactic acid bacteria, 44

lauric acid, 207

lavender, 148

lawn chemicals, 74–75

Ledum, 145

leptospirosis, 204–206

Listeria, 199

liver detox, 115–116

liver function, 77, 109–110, 114

Lyme disease, 204

lymphosarcoma (lymphoma), 104–105, 134

M

Mackerel and Oatmeal, 198

Maddie's story, 12–13

malassezia, 92–95

malvin, 31

mast cells, 34

Mellor, Judith, 43, 184

Merc corr 30c, 156

Mercurius sol, 147

Metronidazole, 155

microbiome, 93

microencapsulation, 170

microorganisms, 42–45

milk thistle, 78

mineral/vitamin supplements. *See* supplements

molecular mimicry, 41, 182

monoclonal antibody therapy (mAb), 87–89

monolaurin, 207

muscle response testing, 176, 177

mycoplasmas, 41, 43, 181–182

mycotoxins, 83

N

Nambudripad, Devi, 174

Nambudripad's Allergy Elimination Technique (NAET), 43, 174–176

natural killer cells (NK), 120

Natural Resources Defense Council (NRDC), 75

natural versus conventional medicine, 163–171

Nellie's story, 9, 178–179

noncore vaccinations

Photo Credits

Front cover: Grigorita Ko/Sshutterstock

Back cover: Peter Wollinga/Shutterstock

Title page: Irina Kozorog/Shutterstock

Contents page: Chendongshan/Shutterstock

Yellow chapter opener graphic, pages 7, 17, 21, 25, 33, 39, 47, 65, 73, 81, 91, 107, 125, 139, 151, 163, 173, 189: Spring Bine/Shutterstock

Dandelion graphic, pages 2, 4-5, 79, 89, 97, 103, 109, 123, 149, 159, 178, 183, 201, 224: Maja81/Shutterstock

Sidebar dog and cat, pages 18, 19, 22, 26, 27, 29, 34, 37, 40, 41, 44, 48, 49, 58, 63, 66, 69, 76, 77, 86, 87, 91, 92, 94, 98, 99, 107, 108, 111, 112, 114, 119, 126, 141, 154, 155, 166, 169, 174, 192, 199, 200, 205,f Susan Schmitz/Shutterstock

About the Author, page 224: Tim Whittaker Photography, Ltd.

Truman, page 9: Deb Kistlern

The following photos courtesy of Shutterstock:

135pixels, 46; 4 PM production, 59 (top); 5 second Studio, 120; Africa Studio, 113, 124, 127, 141; alanisko, 132; Ermolaev Alexander, 8 (top and bottom), 16, 42, 45, 67, 135 (bottom); alexei_tm, 6; AlinaMD, 77; almaje, 148 (top); Tina Andros, 20; Koldunova Anna, 167; anyaivanova, 43; Aprilphoto, 111 (center); Elena Arkadova, 90; aleg baranau, 156; bergamont, 194 (bottom); Billion Photos, 35; Dmitrijs Bindemanis, 94; Boonchuay 1970, 157 (bottom); Javier Brosch, 84; Binh Thanh Bui, 116 (top right); Jayme Burrows, 57; Tony Campbell, 18, 108 ; catinsyrup, 100; Jacek Chabraszewski, 193 (top); vuttichai chaiya, 181; Chendongshan, 38, 116 (bottom), 186; Cherries, 68 (both); Monica Click, 88 (bottom); cynoclub, 13, 111 (bottom); Dionisvera, 135 (top, second from right); Sergei Drozd, 117; Natalia Dvukhimenna, 97; Elnur, 215; EZvereva, 30; Ezzolo, 119; Fabian Faber, 125; February_Love, 146 (inset); K Quinn Ferris, 154; RGallianos, 33; gresei, 193 (bottom); Guzel Studio, 163; Hekla, 142, 177 (top); Lindsay Helms, 152; Pavel Hlystov, 74; JIANG HONGYAN, 144; IMG Stock Studio, 70; inlovepai, 27; Eric Isselee, 21, 29, 47, 52, 82, 86, 89, 105, 160, 166, 210; Brian A Jackson, 22, 168; Jagodka, 54; JetKat, 118; osoznanie.jizni, 135 (top, second from left); JJ IMAGE, 180; Tanya Kalian, 104; kao, 126 (right); Csanad Kiss, 110; Jacqueline Klose, 98; Grigorita Ko, 36, 60, 106; Kateryna Kon, 101; KPG_Payless, 175; kurhan, 199; Artem Kutsenko, 194 (top); Max Lashcheuski, 196 (top); Erik Lam, 170; Emily Li, 28; LianeM, 79; Linda_K, 143; Svetlana Lukienko, 80; Oleksandr Lytvynenko, 176; Viktar Malyshchyts, 201; Cosmin Manci, 65; maoyunping, 174; Marten_House, 123; Mauro Matacchione, 24; Mega Pixel, 193 (center); Nik Merkulov, 128, 129; MindStorm, 31; MirasWonderland, 26; Moving Moments, 194 (center); Myshun, 66; NancyP5, 161; Maks Narodenko, 116 (top left); Mariontxa, 198; Igor

Normann, 25; Chanwit Ohm, 92; Anna Ok, 19, 164; Okeanas, 50; Okssi, 105; BORINA OLGA, 183; Olhastock, 51 (bottom); Sari ONeal, 137; Jarun Ontakarai, 102; Jakkrit Orrasri, 62; oticki, 131 (bottom); otsphoto, 12; pakornkrit, 9 (top), 179; Ronnachai Palas, 88 (top); NIPAPORN PANYACHAROEN, 114 (center); PardoY, 17, 59 (bottom); PeoGeo, 133; Liudmila Pereginskaya, 191; Michael Pettigrew, 4-5, 14, 214; photomaster, 165; Photo-SD, 185; VVadyab Pico, 146; Piyoset, 23; ANURAK PONGPATIMET, 207; Ivan Popovych, 71; PRESSLAB, 48; rangizzz, 153; Ksenia Raykova, 40; Damien Richard, 75; rodimov, 147, 192; Roobcio, 196 (bottom); Rtstudio, 195; Roman Samokhin, 114 (bottom); santypan, 203; Marut Sayannikroth, 32, 138; Susan Schmitz, 64, 73, 112, 126 (left), 139, 177 (bottom); schubbel, 69; Elena Schweitzer, 78; Scorpp, 189; SeaRick1, 34, 158; sematadesign, 56, 209; Kucher Serhii, 93; Oksana Shufrych, 150; Tanya Sid, 134; Angel Simon, 200; Dmitrij Skorobogatov, 121; Sofiaworld, 171; O_Solaro, 44; Olha Solodenko, 140; Alena Stalmashonak, 72; Suti Stock Photo, 173; Gladskikh Tatiana, 87, 136 (top); Joe Thongsan, 95; MR. WICHAI THONGTAPE, 53, 172; Tiger Images, 76, 197; Nikolai Tsvetkov, 85; ALEX_UGALEK, 130; urfin, 51 (top); ViDi Studio, 188; Dmytro Vietrov, 136 (bottom); vipman, 135 (far right); Vivienstock, 109; Hong Vo, 135 (top, far left); Chuck Wagner, 96; Ivonne Wierink, 55; Wisiel, 190; Monika Wisniewska, 205, 213; Peter Wollinga, 83; Kira_Yan, 162; Dora Zett, 39, 145, 148 (bottom); Stephanie Zieber, 41, 131 (top); Suto Norbert Zsolt, 157 (top); Igor Zubkis, 169

About the Author

Dr. Deva K. Khalsa, a licensed doctor of veterinary medicine, earned her VMD degree from the University of Pennsylvania. She is a member of the American Veterinary Medical Association, the American Holistic Veterinary Medical Association, and the International Veterinary Acupuncture Society. She has studied homeopathy for more than thirty years, as well as other alternative therapies, and she lectures nationally and internationally on her fresh and successful approach to veterinary medicine. Her work stems from her belief that animals are at their best and happiest only when they are in a healthy and natural state.

Dr. Khalsa focuses on empowering people to discover and nurture this natural state in their pets and, in doing so, to connect with and celebrate the true spirit of animals. Her best-selling book, *Dr. Khalsa's Natural Dog*, now out in the second edition, is a favorite among veterinarians and dog owners. Visit Dr. Khalsa online at *www.doctordeva.com*.

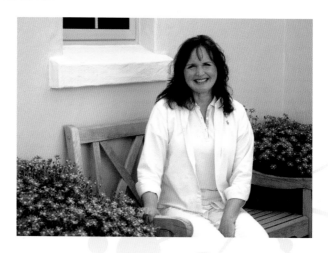